HOT AND BOTHERED

Also by Jancee Dunn

NONFICTION

How Not to Hate Your Husband After Kids

Cyndi Lauper: A Memoir

Why Is My Mother Getting a Tattoo?: And Other Questions I Wish I Never Had to Ask

But Enough About Me: How a Small-Town Girl Went from Shag Carpet to the Red Carpet

FICTION

Don't You Forget About Me

HOT AND BOTHERED

What No One Tells You About Menopause and How to Feel Like Yourself Again

JANCEE DUNN

G. P. PUTNAM'S SONS
NEW YORK

PUTNAM
— EST. 1838 —

G. P. Putnam's Sons
Publishers Since 1838
An imprint of Penguin Random House LLC
penguinrandomhouse.com

Library of Congress Cataloging-in-Publication Data

Names: Dunn, Jancee, author.
Title: Hot and bothered : what no one tells you about menopause and how to feel like yourself again / Jancee Dunn.
Description: New York : G. P. Putnam's Sons, 2023. |
Includes bibliographical references and index.
Identifiers: LCCN 2023004715 (print) | LCCN 2023004716 (ebook) |
ISBN 9780593542569 (hardcover) | ISBN 9780593542576 (ebook)
Subjects: LCSH: Menopause—Popular works.
Classification: LCC RG186.D86 2023 (print) | LCC RG186 (ebook) |
DDC 618.1/75—dc23/eng/20230207
LC record available at https://lccn.loc.gov/2023004715
LC ebook record available at https://lccn.loc.gov/2023004716
p. cm.

Printed in the United States of America
1st Printing

Book design by Tiffany Estreicher

This book aims to provide useful information about menopause that serves as a starting point, but is not intended to replace the diagnostic expertise and medical advice of your doctor. Please consult with your doctor before making any health decisions, particularly if you suffer from any medical conditions that may require treatment.

To Judy Dunn, my mom

• Contents •

Author's Note

The names in this book are real and used with the subjects' permission, except for my own doctor, who asked to be anonymous, and a few friends whose last names are omitted.

While I did my best in my reporting to ensure the accuracy of the medical information presented in this book, I am not a doctor. I am not dispensing medical advice in this book; I am relaying my own story and the treatment options that were presented to me. This book's suggestions are not intended as a substitute for readers consulting with their own doctors to get the best medical care for their own particular needs and situation. (As I'll say many times in the book, every experience with menopause is different.)

A few words about the use of the word *women* in these pages: I use the terms *women* and *female* in the book as shorthand for "people with ovaries" when I am referring to research, but I tried, as much as possible, to use gender-neutral phraseology such as *people* and *partners.* Most people associate menopause with cisgender women, but it can affect people of all genders. Many nonbinary and transgender people experience menopause. Diversity and inclusion are vital in all aspects of menopausal support.

HOT AND BOTHERED

• Chapter 1 •

What to Expect When You're No Longer Expecting

Menopause Is a Condition Shared by Half the Population—So Why Is It Still Spoken of in Whispers?

In the summer of my forty-fifth year, I suddenly found myself lurching awake at three A.M. with the sort of instant alertness that meant hours of sleeplessness lay ahead. Staring into the darkness, I would attempt all the soothing, borderline-monotonous mind tricks I'd recommended as a longtime health writer: progressive stretching exercises, reciting state capitals, planning weekly meals. None worked. In the daytime, I stumbled around, fuzzy and fatigued, trying to keep pace with my toddler.

One supposedly effective method to bring on slumber is to take a mental tour of your childhood home. And so, on one fidgety night, I visited my former house in Pittsburgh, last seen in 1975. Here was the avocado-colored fridge in the kitchen; there was the brown plaid couch that sagged in the middle. By the couch sat a fake-wood side table, which contained, in true seventies style, an embedded metal ashtray. When my parents finished huffing a Kool, they would push a button on top of the ashtray, which spun the ashes and butts into a mottled collection bin below, where the smoky mulch remained for months.

Why didn't my parents empty the reeking table ashtray? I wondered one night. Maybe they were somehow comforted by the smell of old cigarette butts? The ashtrays in our light-blue Buick LeSabre were always filled to overflowing, too. When did cars start phasing out ashtrays and cigarette lighters?

My meandering thoughts were narcotizing enough, yet I still couldn't drop off. What the hell was wrong with me? I had never had sleep problems in my life. I turned over, careful not to wake my husband or jostle my boobs, which had been sore lately.

I froze. *My boobs, which had been sore lately.*

Hold up. When was my last period? I calculated backward. Two months. I had gone off the Pill the year before, but we practiced the horribly named "rhythm method," in which we avoided sex during my supposedly fertile times.

My blood chilled further as I realized I was bloated, too. "Tom," I whispered. It was nearly dawn, anyway, and our two-year-old daughter would be awake soon. He opened his eyes blearily; as I told him my suspicions, he abruptly sat up. We had always wanted one child, and we were content with our choice. We had never even considered another. Nor was I young: I'd given birth to Sylvie the week before my forty-third birthday, after a so-called geriatric pregnancy. I did not envision myself as a forty-five-year-old (soon to be forty-six-year-old) parent to another newborn. I had already developed lower back problems from lifting our kid.

Tom and I sat quietly in bed, our heads whirling with the emotional, financial, and logistical complications of having another child.

Finally he reached over and squeezed my hand. "If this turns out to be a pregnancy, well, then . . ." He broke off, then gathered himself. "Well then, we'll make it work."

I covered his hand with mine. "I was thinking the same thing," I said in a high, choked voice.

• • • •

I wasn't pregnant.

I had skipped my periods because I was perimenopausal.

I know this now, but I didn't then. Because I was in my mid-forties, the idea of perimenopause—the term for the transition into menopause, *peri* meaning *around*—simply hadn't occurred to me. I was taking my toddler to Elmo-themed birthday parties. I still had my childhood teddy bear. I bought my pajamas from teen websites because they were cheaper (I just avoided the crop tops). I had a vague idea that menopause awaited, hazily, in the future—but that was still far off, when I'd start wearing visor hats and orthopedic food-service clogs. Wasn't menopause for, you know, older ladies? It had always been an easy subject to stash away.

Soon after, my periods grew more erratic: a drought one month, the Rio Grande the next. Perimenopause lasts, on average, for four years, but it can stretch to eight. Symptoms can sneak up on you—and before you're fully aware, they become your new normal. My nails took on a flaky, baklava-like texture. My mouth became so dry that I began hacking like my hairball-prone cat.

One night I woke up drenched from head to toe. Immediately, I assumed I had peed the bed. When you're a former bedwetter, you never quite outgrow that feeling of *Oh, Lord, I did it again*. My last incident had been in high school, when I'd received a coveted invitation to a sleepover at Kim Johnson's house. Every moment of that night is etched upon my brain. First we watched a *Love Boat* episode starring Sherman Hemsley and Jaclyn Smith while guzzling can after can of grape Shasta. When it was time for bed, Kim's older brother, Raymond, commandeered their one bathroom for what seemed like hours. (*What could he be doing in there?* I remember thinking naively.) Eventually, as I nervously waited in one of Kim's twin beds for Raymond to leave, I fell asleep.

Later that night, I was horrified to discover that I had duly peed Kim's bed. This would be all over the school Monday morning unless I acted quickly. While Kim slept, I stealthily removed the fitted sheet, fanned it up and down for an hour until it was dry, then, slowly and quietly, turned the mattress over and replaced the sheet.

Kim never knew.

I had the same feeling of dread as I lay stuck to my sheets. Why did I swig so much lemonade last night? Did the pee reach my sleeping husband?

Tom heard me stirring, turned over, and stared, confused, at my wet hair, which was plastered to my head. "Did you just work out?" he said, squinting at me.

No, I told him. Nor, I eventually figured out, had I peed myself. It was night sweats.

Peeing myself was still ahead.

• • • •

At my annual physical a few months later, I mentioned the night sweats to my doctor, who ran a battery of fruitless tests and briskly concluded that it was probably "stress." This conveniently vague quasi diagnosis was not exactly wrong—who *doesn't* have stress?—but is used, research shows, more often on female patients. As the months rolled on and my symptoms piled up, I saw a dentist for my bleeding gums, a dermatologist for my crawlingly itchy skin, a cardiologist for my irregular heartbeat. After spending countless hours

"In my adult life, I don't
recall one serious conversation
with another woman about
what to expect."

—Oprah Winfrey

in doctors' waiting rooms, I had caught up on all the latest issues of *Reader's Digest* but was no closer to any sort of prognosis. Not one of them connected my symptoms to menopause.

My experience was not exactly novel: perimenopausal women can spend several years trying to get the right diagnosis and treatment. Medicine, of course, has a long history of telling women that their symptoms are all in their heads; it's even more common, studies have found, for women of color and those of larger size.

When I finally figured out what was happening to my body and brain, I was floored. How could I have been so clueless? I'm a health writer, for god's sake. For more than two decades, I've been reporting on mental and physical health for publications such as *The New York Times*, *Vogue*, and *O, The Oprah Magazine*. I had a longtime sex column in *GQ*. I've written countless articles about women's health, and have interviewed hundreds of physicians and scientists over the years. As a patient, I diligently schedule all my annual "well visits" on the first week of January. I am what doctors would term a "well-informed, active self-manager of my medical care." How is it that I never had a single conversation with anybody about a life transition that lasts for years, sometimes a decade plus?

And if I was unprepared, what about all the women who *don't* write about health for a living? I tell Makeba Williams, MD, vice chair of professional development and wellness and associate professor of obstetrics and gynecology at Washington University School of Medicine in Saint Louis, how mortified I am that I didn't pick up on this.

"Oh, you can't believe the bewilderment that I encounter on a daily basis," says Williams, a certified menopause practitioner. "Menopause is so little talked about as a transition in our lives that it really catches people off guard. So they come in blindsided, having no understanding that many of these changes that they're experiencing are related to a normal, natural physiologic event. Or they've been grossly misinformed, and I sort of have to bring them back and reset." She sighs. "We haven't done the anticipatory guidance to prepare women. We have to create expectations around menopause and normalize it, just like we do for puberty."

"Hey, I'm in D.C., where you've got some of the smartest, wealthiest people on the planet," chimes in urologist and sexual medicine specialist Rachel S. Rubin, MD, assistant clinical professor at Georgetown University Hospital and owner of a sexual medicine private practice, "and they are fucking clueless."

Certainly my mother, who gritted through the Change in silence, never said a single word to me about it. We have coming-of-age ceremonies for girls who are becoming women, such as the Jewish bat mitzvah, and celebratory rituals, such as wedding and baby showers, where vital information is exchanged to help prepare the person to enter the next realm of life. There's no menopause shower, where a woman is given gifts like neck cream, portable fans, and vaginal lube. When it comes to menopause, no one sits you down for the Talk.

That includes many doctors. A 2013 survey found that fewer than one in five ob-gyn residents received any formal menopause training at all. Not until 1993 were women and minorities federally mandated to be included in clinical trials.

And don't think that physicians who specialize in women's health get any more insight into this phenomenon. A 2019 survey of internal medicine and ob-gyn residents found that only 6.8 percent felt "adequately prepared" to manage women experiencing menopause.

Back in the day, menopause used to be the domain of gynecologists, but as the 2013 survey coauthor Wen Shen, MD, associate professor in the Johns Hopkins Medicine Department of Gynecology and Obstetrics in Baltimore, tells me, things have changed.

"Traditionally, gynecology has been a procedure/surgical specialty, and insurance companies reimburse well for procedures," says Shen. (To put this in perspective, according to the nonprofit FAIR Health, the national average cost for an obstetrician to deliver a baby vaginally in 2018 was $12,290.) "During the menopause transition especially, many significant health changes take place in women, and clinical care for these women requires time-intensive counseling," Shen continues. "And reimbursement for time spent with a patient to promote healthy aging and preventive medicine is less well-paid."

My friend Mira, who realized she had gone a year without her period, booked an appointment with her ob-gyn to figure out what to do next. After a few desultory questions, her ob-gyn handed her a pamphlet on menopause, suggested she take up yoga, and hustled her out the door. "She wasn't being dismissive," says Mira. "I just think she didn't know what to tell me."

Lauren Streicher is a professor of obstetrics and gynecology at Northwestern University Feinberg School of Medicine. "I give the students the lecture on female sexual function and dysfunction," she says. "They have four years of medical school. My lecture's the only one on this subject, and I get twenty minutes. Oh, and it's optional. Twenty minutes of an optional lecture! I talk very fast."

Even if women know what symptoms to look for and actually seek treatment, a Yale School of Medicine study found that they aren't likely to get it. Researchers looked at insurance claims from 500,000 women and found that three-quarters of the women who sought medical attention for their menopause symptoms got no treatment at all. A 2021 AARP survey of women age thirty-five and up found that only 18 percent said they felt "very informed" about what to expect in menopause and perimenopause.

In other words, 82 percent of us are walking around largely oblivious about the most significant change in our physical lives since puberty.

When I started researching the symptoms myself, I almost wished I had stayed clueless. The literature bristles with words like *atrophy*, *deterioration*, and *withered*. You are confronted by phrases like *significant loss of breast volume* and *having less sex* and *the menopausal rats showed higher levels of anxiety.*

Here is a description of the multiple forms of menopausal urinary incontinence:

> *As the tissues of your vagina and urethra lose elasticity, you may experience frequent, sudden, strong urges to urinate, followed by an involuntary loss of urine (urge incontinence), or the loss of urine with coughing, laughing, or lifting (stress incontinence).*

If I was "laughing," it was only so as not to cry. When I first read this, I went from being a reasonably vibrant woman in what I thought was my prime to envisioning the short remainder of my life as a grim, relentless trudge, in my food-service clogs and wash 'n' go hairdo, right into an open grave.

• • • •

In the years during which I transitioned into menopause, I churned through many doctors, not just because my symptoms were a mystery, but my finances as a freelance writer varied wildly from year to year. As a result, my health plans were perpetually changing, prompting me to constantly recruit a fresh round of physicians.

Some were wonderful. Others were as dismissive as Mira's yoga-loving ob-gyn. When I asked one primary care physician about the sudden weight gain around my middle, he patted his own stomach and chuckled. "That's just middle age!" he said cheerily. I left feeling unsettled. I was supposed to shrug at my sudden stomach bulge? What if it was a tumor?

Many eminent menopause specialists offer similar stories of flummoxed patients who notice symptoms and immediately imagine something dire. "I have women come in every year with achiness, a really common symptom, and they've seen two or three rheumatologists and think they have Lyme disease," says Mary Jane Minkin, a clinical professor in the Department of Obstetrics, Gynecology, and Reproductive Sciences at the Yale University School of Medicine. "A lot of them also get palpitations and think they have heart disease."

Assuming the worst is an ongoing theme in menopause chat rooms. In one that I now lurk in, phrases like *Am I dying?* and *I'm afraid I'm dying* are heartbreakingly common; in post after post, people write of menopause-related panic attacks that send them racing to the emergency room, convinced it's a coronary or a stroke. Why is information about this process, which affects half the earth's population, so difficult to find? Many experts have told me that menopause treatment is the biggest gap in women's healthcare in the United States.

Even if a woman is aware that she's in perimenopause or menopause, the burden is typically on *her* to find ways to deal with it. In a perimenopause chat room, as the participants swapped tips, they sounded variously like psychopharmacologists, In Goop Health summit attendees, and Big Mikey, my ex-boyfriend's drug dealer:

> *Magnesium, calcium, and vitamin D supplements helped me with stress. Melatonin 1.5 grams a night, 350 mg magnesium ci-*

trate, but you can start with 650 mg the first week—caution, you will notice loose stools if you continue with the higher dose of magnesium. Rhubarb root, EMDR [eye movement desensitization and reprocessing] therapy, Lunesta, 3 mg. For insomnia, I take edibles with THC. Prozac and acupuncture helped so much with the sadness and physical issues. Antidepressants and weed, just to get you over the hump.

When I first read these tips, they all sounded so extreme. Now none of them do.

• • • •

Menopause! The very word sets people on edge. The M word has been referred to, seemingly in whispers, as far back as the Bible. In a passage from Genesis, Abraham's wife Sarah is described as "advanced in age; it had ceased to be with Sarah after the manner of women." You can almost hear the writer casting around for some sort of euphemism: *She had, er, you know . . . "it had ceased to be."*

Some physicians in ancient times believed that older women's wombs wandered restlessly around the body, like I do around my house, in search of my "readers." The second-century AD physician Aretaeus of Cappadocia claimed that a woman's womb "moved of itself hither and thither."

Fortunately, it was easy enough to bring the meandering womb to heel. The womb, wrote Aretaeus, "delights in fragrant smells, and advances toward them, and it had an aversion to fetid smells, and flees from them, and on the whole is like an animal within an animal."

As Helen King wrote in *Hysteria Beyond Freud*, the fifth-century BCE Greek physician Hippocrates, known as the father of modern medicine, theorized that the uterus in widows is unsatisfied and not only produces toxic fumes but also takes to roaming around the body, in search not of "fragrant smells" but of moisture. It seems the liver was one stop on the womb's peregrinations. As King writes, Hippocrates believed that "if a woman's vessels are emptier than usual and she is more tired, the womb, dried out by fatigue, turns around and 'throws itself' on the liver because this organ is full of moisture."

Descriptions of a woman's worn-out reproductive organs could be merciless. In her book *The Woman in the Body: A Cultural Analysis of Reproduction*, anthropologist Emily Martin unearthed this description of Ceasing to Be from an early medical textbook: "The *senile ovary* is a shrunken and puckered organ, containing few if any follicles, and made up for the most part of . . . the bleached and functionless remainders of corpora lutea." This sounds like the dismal prognosis of a marine biologist surveying the Great Barrier Reef after the effects of climate change.

If we continue with the nautical theme, Victorian doctors believed, according to the authors of *The Curse: A Cultural History of Menstruation*, that women grew scales on their breasts after they stopped menstruating. (Given the state of my newly desiccated skin, they weren't entirely off the mark.)

Menopause was given a formal name in the 1820s, as Susan Mattern writes in *The Slow Moon Climbs: The Science, History, and Meaning of Menopause,* from a combination of *menos,* the Greek word for month, and *pausie*, Greek for cessation. We can thank a nineteenth-century French physician named Dr. Charles de Gardanne for the nomenclature. And while he deserves credit for at least naming the transition, Mattern goes on, he also cited fifty conditions for which menopause was responsible, including scurvy, gout, and nymphomania.

In the nineteenth and early twentieth centuries, doctors attempted various "cures" for menopause. Dr. Andrew F. Currier, author of the 1897 book *The Menopause; A Consideration of the Phenomena Which Occur to Women at the Close of the Child-Bearing Period*, suggested that menopausal women purge their bowels with saline solution ("the bowels should be kept freely open, as such people are in very many instances constipated"). One symptom that accompanied menopause that Currier mentioned was "nervous pain"—what we would today call anxiety. (He wasn't necessarily wrong. Anxiety is one of the thirty-four various symptoms doctors have identified in menopausal women—more on that soon.) For "nervous pain," he suggested tampons soaked in glycerin and silver nitrate, or bleeding from incisions in the arms or legs.

Currier emphasized that menopausal symptoms only affected certain types of women. "Among the degraded, and among those, too, who are subject to the vicissitudes of out-of-door life and manual labor, the menopause is least likely to excite attention or create disturbance," Currier wrote-slash-mansplained. "It is among the highly bred, tenderly reared women of civilized life, that the menopause is a matter of great significance." While many among "the degraded" may have vociferously disagreed with Currier, then, as now, the usual portrayal of a menopausal woman excludes low-income and working-class people—as well as LGBTQIA+ people, and people of color.

Alexander Hubert Providence Leuf, meanwhile, in his 1902 tome *Gynecology, Obstetrics, Menopause*, offered an alarming prescription for night sweats: a tincture of 5 to 20 drops of belladonna, a poisonous plant also known as deadly nightshade. For constipation, due to menopausal women's "dulled sensibility of the bowels," he suggested a bracing, neurotoxic purge of *mercury*.

In the nineteenth century, writes health sciences professor Elizabeth Siegel Watkins in *The Estrogen Elixir*, doctors gave patients products containing animal ovaries to treat various conditions related to "ovarian failure," such as the ever-popular hysteria. Women were prescribed solutions of ovarian extract in water, while others who were perhaps more into whole foods were told to eat "fresh sow or cow ovaries, minced and served in sandwiches." (Mustard or mayo was presumably optional.) In the 1890s, writes Thom Rooke in *The Quest for Cortisone*, Merck & Company rolled out the first hormonal product marketed for menopause, called Ovariin, a coarse brownish powder made of dried and pulverized cow ovaries. At least it was available in vanilla flavor. ("It's hard to imagine that pulverized cow ovaries didn't already taste great without the extra flavoring," Rooke notes.)

American biochemist and Nobel Prize winner Edward Doisy isolated estrogen in 1929. A decade later, a commercial product for menopause made from the urine of a pregnant mare was introduced. It was called, with admirable transparency, Premarin. One memorable vintage Premarin ad showed a photo of a fed-up bus driver. *He is suffering from estrogen deficiency*, read the caption. On the other side is an agitated female passenger of a certain age. *She is the reason why* is inscribed below her angry face. Menopause was seen as a problem—*for men*.

My favorite Premarin ad, from the 1970s, shows a worried-looking middle-aged man with reading glasses who clutches a newspaper; he is flanked by two cowering adult children. In the foreground is an older woman, holding her forehead. *Almost any tranquilizer might calm her down* . . . reads the copy . . . *but at her age, estrogen may be what she really needs*. The makers hedged their bets, however: one version of Premarin was laced with phenobarbital, a powerfully addictive drug used for anxiety and "seizure control."

an exam and sort of peering in there and saying, 'Oh, well, your ovaries are dried up now.'" She laughs.

After he put her on Premarin, "it really helped with my red-faced sweats and the hot flashes and made me feel less like tearing someone's hair off," she says. "The gynecologist said it also helped with strengthening bones. It was a pill that came in a round case, and you just clicked it around to the next day. It was very easy."

I ask her how old she was when she stopped taking Premarin and she thinks a minute. "I honestly can't remember," she says finally. "Some news started coming out that it was not good for you. It's not like you could google information like you do now. You just sort of trusted that it was right. But I'll tell you something, I wish I had continued it, because my hot flashes, especially at night, lasted for years. Years!"

As I help her load roses into a cart, I ask her if she had the Premarin with phenobarbital. "Is that the stuff that knocks you out?" She considered. "Hm. Maybe. I don't remember. Sounds like a good idea, though." Mom likes her sleeping pills.

• • • •

It's not just that the drugs and treatments available for women in menopause were absurd and barbaric (although they were). It's also that they were largely untested—if women were even invited to be part of the medical conversation at all.

Even after Dr. Doisy had isolated estrogen in the 1920s, research on women's health in the twentieth century was scant (and research on menopausal women of color is still gallingly rare). In the early sixties, after researchers noticed that women tended to have lower rates of heart disease until menopause, when their estrogen levels dropped, they conducted the first trial to see whether estrogen supplements were an effective preventive treatment. The study, published in 1973, was conducted on 8,341 men. And zero women.

The treatment of menopause is "an utter disaster," says Rachel Rubin of Georgetown University Hospital. A woman's quality of life during menopause is almost never discussed, she adds. "I'm a urologist who treats all genders, and we care so much about how men are urinating, their sexual function, their libido, their erections. We love talking about quality of life. That is not in any kind of conversation we're having around women. We never lead with quality of life. We are always talking about risk reducing. Will this kill you, will you get cancer, will this hurt the baby?" She sighs. "We do not talk about quality of life in women enough. We don't even have the vocabulary to do that."

Instead, she says, "The messaging is, 'This is aging, just pick yourself up by your bootstraps! You're a woman, just try harder! Meditate! Exercise more! Why aren't you exercising more?' We, as a society, don't do a great job of saying, 'Okay, that's a biological condition that doesn't feel so good. And maybe there are biological solutions.'"

Fear of menopause, writes British historian Louise Foxcroft in *Hot Flushes, Cold Science: A History of the Modern Menopause*, "is something we have learned, and it has grown out of a general, male, and medical distaste for the idea of the menopause perceived as an end of viability, fertility, beauty, desirability, and worth." (In the UK, it's called *hot flushes* and *the menopause.*) In our youth-centric society, if your eggs are past their sell-by date, off you go to the clearance shelf!

In a now-famous episode of *Inside Amy Schumer*, Schumer happens upon a festive, wine-filled picnic in the woods with Patricia Arquette, Tina Fey, and Julia-Louis Dreyfuss. They are celebrating

Louis-Dreyfuss's so-called "last fuckable day"—the time in every actress's life, as Louis-Dreyfuss cheerfully explains, when "the media decides you finally reach the point where you're not believably fuckable anymore."

As they tip back more wine, Arquette shares that she didn't get a commercial she auditioned for because the director deemed her "too old to play Larry King's wife." Then they all discover that they read for the film part of Mrs. Claus. ("Hey, who got that?" "J. Lo." "Oh, she'll be good.") When Schumer asks if men have a last fuckable day, they all laugh merrily and say no—even if, says Fey, they're one hundred and ejaculating "nothing but white spiders."

For the most part, cultural squeamishness around what some doctors term "reverse puberty" remains rampant. Jill Angelo, founder of a Seattle company that provides telemedicine for women in menopause, tells me she once met with potential investors and one worriedly asked her about menopause's "ick factor." Fear of menopause is also based on the unknown, says Hadine Joffe, Paula A. Johnson Professor of Psychiatry in the Field of Women's Health at Harvard Medical School. "Which I get, because people know so little about it, and they have no idea what it is. So a lot of their associations and their projections onto it are negative."

Type "pregnancy" in Google images, says Joffe, "and the images that come up are lovely and sweet." But if you Google "menopause," she says, there is nothing about a normal life transition. "Instead, it's all symptom-based and problem-based. It's not about a midlife process, it's always this kind of angry tone, about being irritable and sleepless. Why is it that the first association with menopause is all these problems? Some people go through it and never have problems."

"Oh, I'm constantly on my soapbox about how the world has ignored menopause—an experience that affects every single woman who lives into midlife," says Pauline Maki, a professor of psychiatry, psychology, and obstetrics and gynecology at the University of Illinois at Chicago College of Medicine and past president of the North American Menopause Society. "And it ticks me off because it's ageist and sexist."

As a urologist, Dr. Rubin has an easy way to help her male patients grasp what menopause is about. "I tell them, 'You want to know what menopause feels like? All we have to do is cut your testicles off. And guess what the side effects are? Hot flashes. Night sweats. Brain fog. Depression. Cardiovascular disease. Low libido. Erectile dysfunction. *That's* menopause.'"

Portrayals of menopause on social media are largely not positive, adds Dr. Rubin. "I always say that menopause has the worst PR campaign in the history of the universe," she says. When it comes to branding this phase of life or getting positive messages out there to combat the negative stereotypes about women's lives in midlife, "we're not winning on social media."

There are currently around 30 million U.S. women aged forty to fifty-four in the United States. Why are we so unprepared for one of the most monumental transitions of our lives? It affects family, friends, and coworkers. It affects the nonbinary and the transgendered. Not every woman goes through childbirth—birth rates have been dropping in the United States for years, and a 2021 report by the U.S. Census Bureau found that nearly one in six adults over fifty-five are child-free. But all women, if they live long enough, will go through menopause. It's an experience shared by half the population . . . only no one is sharing.

If the average age of menopause is fifty-one and the average life expectancy of a woman in the United States is eighty, she will spend a third of her life in menopause. You don't "go through" menopause; you enter it and you stay there.

"It's not like opening and closing the door," says Lubna Pal, professor of obstetrics, gynecology, and reproductive sciences and director of the Menopause Program at Yale School of Medicine. "It's a pathway. It's not a disease. It's not a disorder. It's a phase of life."

The manifesto from Beatrice Dixon, founder in 2014 of The Honey Pot Company, a plant-based line of feminine care products made "by humans with vaginas for humans with vaginas," is even more delightfully blunt: "A lot of times we feel like we're the only person going through this, but what pulls us together is that we're all going through the same shit at the same time! How can something be taboo when we're all going through it?"

Dixon says that if anyone is squeamish in product meetings—say, about the Honey Pot's line of incontinence pads and liners "to liberate you from the dribble," one of the leading symptoms of menopause—Dixon quickly sets them straight. "If I hear, 'Uh, I don't necessarily want to have this conversation about incontinence,' well, I'm not the person to talk to if you don't want to talk about real shit," she says. "I try to remind them quickly that everyone on this planet came from a vagina. When and if those silly things present themselves, that's the place that I typically go to."

Which is why we need to stop talking about menopause in whispers, says Dixon. "Age, hormonal imbalances, any condition, it's all natural and normal and there is nothing new under the sun," she says. "Shame, guilt—you don't have time for that shit."

Dixon is correct: we don't have time for that shit. By 2025, according to an oft-cited statistic from the North American Menopause Society, more than a billion women around the world will be postmenopausal. It's time to recognize, and normalize, this life transition. Let's go.

• Chapter 2 •

Why Didn't I Know This?

Many of Us Get "The Talk" for Our First Period. No One Gets It for Our Last One.

Of the purported thirty-four symptoms of perimenopause and menopause, some border on surreal.

Aside from the more familiar hot flashes, night sweats, and irregular periods, they are as follows: mood swings, plummeting libido, breast soreness, headaches, vaginal dryness, burning mouth, tingling in hands and feet, gum disease, extreme fatigue, bloating, digestive problems, joint pain, depression, muscle aches, itchy skin, electric shocks, terrible sleep, brain fog, memory lapses, thinning hair, brittle nails, weight gain (five pounds on average, certainly more in my case) incontinence, dizziness or vertigo, increased allergies, loss of bone density, irregular heartbeat, weird new body odor, irritability, anxiety, and panic disorder.

Dryness is a recurring theme, which, in my case, tracked: Everything on my body that was capable of becoming parched did so, from scalp to feet. Even my ears, normally fairly supple as far as ears go, assumed the precise leathery texture of Trader Joe's unsulfured Just Mango Slices. My suddenly dry neck shed so much skin that my white towels turned brown (perimenopausal sisters, I implore you to switch, this minute, to a rich neck cream).

My nether regions experienced a calamitous climate change, swiftly going from Tropical Lush to Arid Desert. Sex with my husband felt like he had strapped on a condom made of Astroturf. The hair on my head not only thinned but seemingly migrated down my body to sprout in unwelcome WTF places, such as my inner wrist.

And yes, sudden, strange BO hijacked my body. It was the acrid chemical tang that arose from wearing a polyester shirt all day in August, with middle notes of Wet Dog, and sweetish top notes of Gas Station Trash Can. It surfaced no matter how recently I had bathed or how heavily I doused my pits with deodorant. (According to the Cleveland Clinic, hormonal fluctuations can indeed change your body's scent, including that of your vagina, and yes, it's normal.)

I ask Mary Jane Minkin of Yale School of Medicine if the oft-repeated "thirty-four symptoms of menopause" is, in her many decades of clinical experience, correct. She considers for a minute. "Yeah, that sounds about right," she says.

I am visiting the eminent ob-gyn at her office at Yale on a blustery fall morning. Minkin, as disarming as she is brilliant, is delightfully down to earth ("crap," it soon becomes clear, is one of her favorite words). She greets me in a crisp white coat and oversize black glasses, and ushers me to a chair with her characteristic vigor. I tell her that when I skipped a period, I fully assumed I was pregnant, and she nods. "I personally have delivered three forty-seven-year-olds who were not trying to get pregnant, believe me." One of

“Literally it was like somebody put a furnace in my core, and turned it on high, and then everything started melting. I thought, ‘Well, this is crazy. I can’t do this.’”

—Michelle Obama on the hot flashes she experienced aboard Marine One them, she goes on, found out, to her shock, that not only was she pregnant, but that the baby was due on the day her daughter was getting married. "They ended up postponing the wedding for a month so the baby could come," she says, shaking her head. "I don't make this stuff up."

I ask Minkin about some of the lesser-known symptoms of menopause, such as joint pain. "Right," she says, nodding. "Joint pain presents similar to fibromyalgia. It can just be this miserable achiness, and women don't know why it's happening. Sometimes they've seen a bunch of rheumatologists. I think the lining of the joint, sometimes referred to as the synovial membrane, gets dry, and the estrogen helps lubricate that lining, kind of like greasing the hinges on a door. I tell these patients they should consider a round of estrogen therapy."

Many women also report that they experience formication, the unwelcome sensation often described as having bugs crawling all over your skin (*forma* is Latin for ant). Which is decidedly unpleasant, whether the bugs are real or imagined.

Others swear that their voices are getting lower or more "gravelly." As it turns out, this is not their imagination. Research shows that the dropping levels of estrogen and progesterone have an effect on the function of a woman's vocal cords, says Abdul-Latif Hamdan, MD, professor of otolaryngology, head and neck surgery at the American University of Beirut, and founder of the Hamdan Voice Unit. This results, he says, in an array of symptoms often referred to as postmenopausal vocal syndrome, or PMVS, including vocal fatigue, loss of range, inability to reach the high notes, deepening of the voice, and throat clearing.

Happily, he has also found in his research, and that of others, that menopausal hormone therapy can reverse some of these symptoms, including lower pitch, "simply by restoring the hormonal profile that women had before menopause," he says. If you've ever wondered how some female singers in midlife and beyond are able to hit the high notes, while your grandma sounds more and more like James Earl Jones, they may very well be on hormone therapy. English opera singer Lesley Garrett, a soprano, credits hormone therapy for saving her soprano and her career. (An opera singer can't get away with using Auto-Tune.)

• • • •

Not only does menopause affect all women differently, but emerging research shows that symptoms vary, sometimes dramatically, across ethnicities. The pioneering Study of Women's Health Across the Nation (SWAN), which has been following a cohort of U.S. Black, white, Chinese, Japanese, and Hispanic women in midlife since 1994, has uncovered all kinds of disparities.

A 2022 SWAN study found that Black women encountered more episodes of depression and interrupted sleep than white women during the menopause transition and were *less* likely to receive treatment. Meanwhile, Latina women, the researchers found, experience more vaginal dryness and urine leakage than other women.

According to research presented at a 2021 American Heart Association meeting, Black women are also three times more likely to undergo premature menopause (menopause before the age of forty), leading to a 40 percent greater risk of developing coronary heart disease later on. While our physiology may be the same, our experiences are not.

Many experiences of puberty and "reverse puberty" are the same: crying jags, insecurity, mood swings, zits, unexpected changes on your body. (I've been retreating to my bedroom to blast music as I did when I was a teen, although I no longer write "this town SUX" in my diary.)

Some things are markedly different: During puberty, teens feel like everyone is watching them. Menopausal women often feel that no one is. Also, by the time symptoms show up, we're old enough that we suspect that this could be the end.

Not every woman, it should be pointed out, will endure symptoms. The best-case scenario, Minkin tells me, is that she simply stops having periods for a year and feels perfectly normal. "Twenty percent of women will never get one hot flash," Minkin says.

Nor are all symptoms bleak. "Here's something," she offers cheerfully. "Fibroids often shrink during the menopause transition because of the reduction in the estrogen that usually feeds them."

Her Yale colleague Lubna Pal stops by Minkin's office with a mug of tea. "Also, menstruation is not really a joy, is it?" she adds dryly. We all laugh.

• • • •

Thanks to the ageism and sexism that have infused every discussion of this topic (and, let's be frank, of our lives), no one quite knows where to put menopause in our current culture.

In popular music, it's virtually invisible, except to sometimes serve as a generic insult, as in Snoop Dogg's "Upside Down," in which he threatens to treat a rival "like an old bitch and menopause him." A rare exception is Prince's relatively thoughtful offer in "Jack U Off": "I only do it for a worthy cause / Virginity or menopause, you'll have / an instant heart attack if I jack u off." (Who was more qualified than the Purple One to alleviate vaginal atrophy?)

On television, menopause is usually the subject of snickering jokes, but there have been a few exceptions. In 1972, the sitcom *All in the Family* broke ground with an episode titled "Edith's Problem," where she talked about feeling like she's "jumpin' in and out of a hot bath and somebody's twisting a rubber band around my head."

When her daughter explains that it's "the change," Edith's husband, Archie, bellows to his wife that he's going to give her thirty seconds to do it. While the episode, which won an Emmy, seems very ham-fisted now, it was revolutionary at a time when menopause wasn't discussed in public, writes TV critic David Mello. "But *All in the Family* took a sledgehammer to that social barrier and the episode will live on forever because of it."

In 1990, *The Cosby Show's* Clair Huxtable tells her children, in a refreshingly straightforward way, that she is beginning menopause. Her kids freak out, so she pranks them by exaggerating her symptoms. ("A person could burn up in this room," she yells as she runs to the freezer, opens the door, and thrusts her head in.) Eventually she fesses up.

In the past few years, some shows, notably created by women, have inched closer to more fundamental truths. In a now-famous monologue from a 2019 episode of *Fleabag*, Belinda, played by Kristin Scott Thomas, tells Fleabag, "Women are born with pain built in. It's our physical destiny: period pain, sore boobs, childbirth. We have pain on a cycle for years and years and years—and then, just when you feel that you're making peace with it all, what happens? The fucking menopause comes. And it is *the most* wonderful fucking thing in the world. And yes, your entire pelvic floor crumbles, and you get fucking hot and no one cares, but then? You're free. You're no longer a machine, with parts."

Fleabag breaks in to say that she was told it was horrendous. "It is horrendous," proclaims Belinda. "But then it's magnificent."

That sums up my experience perfectly. Belinda is describing what anthropologist Margaret Mead called postmenopausal zest—that exhilarating feeling of coming into your own. It goes beyond the sweet liberation from buying tampons and the relentless fear of becoming pregnant. It's the freedom from the "disease to please." I find it's, indeed, magnificent to feel self-assured, to be less frightened of risk, to claim time and space for yourself without apology.

In the 2021 miniseries *Nine Perfect Strangers,* Melissa McCarthy plays Frances Welty, a bestselling novelist in midlife. When Frances first meets love interest Tony, played by Bobby Cannavale, she tells him she is having a hot flash—and he recommends progesterone. Even a few years ago, a man and woman having a conversation about menopausal hormone therapy as meet-cute banter would be unthinkable.

Shows devoted to perimenopause are even rarer. One exception is a 2022 episode of *Black-ish,* in which Tracee Ellis Ross's character, Rainbow, is going through perimenopause. "I'm trying to manage this perimenopause and I'm so over it," she says. "I ran for three miles after an ice cream truck today and then I punched a dent into the side of it because they told me they didn't have any more tutti-frutti."

Her mother-in-law, Ruby, tells her it's not so bad. "All of this is yours again," she says, gesturing to Rainbow's body. "And you can finally ask yourself, what does Rainbow Johnson want to do? It's your time."

Ruby is right.

• • • •

Let us, as David Bowie once sang, turn and face the strange. We should start with what, precisely, is occurring during the Change.

Most female animals reproduce throughout their life span. But when it comes to humans, the ovaries, compared to other organs, age dramatically and quickly—even as our life spans are stretching further and further out.

Over the last 150 years, according to Eric Verdin, CEO of the Buck Institute, a biomedical institute dedicated to research on aging, our life span has increased two years every decade. This means that we've gone from an average life span of thirty-eight in 1850 to the current life span of seventy-nine to eighty—nearly double.

Why, then, do female humans outlive their fertile period by many decades, while septuagenarian male rock stars are still running around fathering babies?

Both men and women experience age-related hormonal declines. Women's estrogen and progesterone levels can zigzag during perimenopause, drop sharply during menopause, and dwindle to very little postmenopause. Men's testosterone levels, meanwhile, fade away gradually as they age—the decline is steady at around 1 to 2 percent a year from about the age of forty.

This is why the concept of "male menopause," a nonmedical term conjured up by journalists, rankles so many doctors. "The notion of 'male menopause,' a supposed syndrome of male hormone decline associated with aging, shows little sign of life," a 2007 editorial in the medical journal *Menopause* asserted. You can practically see the eye roll implied with the authors' quotes around the term *male menopause*. "It is now time for a decent burial."

Why the disparity in age-related hormonal changes? Evolutionary biologists have been trying to figure this out for over a half century.

One leading idea, first proposed in the 1960s, is called the grandmother hypothesis. (This was also the answer to a disturbingly worded 2022 *Jeopardy!* question that began *Why don't women die at menopause*?) It posits that human females live well past their reproductive prime because of the benefits they offer to their grandkids, such as providing food and care to the next generation. Tend-ing to children who are already born, the theory goes, may be a better evolutionary investment than a birth, which can be riskier.

How, then, do you know when you've well and truly lost the ability to reproduce and the cafeteria is, in effect, closed? Menopause is the point at which twelve full months have passed since a woman's final menstrual period, or FMP, and the walnut-sized ovaries stop releasing eggs. Sometimes it is triggered by chemotherapy, which can cause enough damage to the ovaries to bring on menopause.

It can also be brought about by certain surgeries. Surgical menopause is menopause that's induced by a medical treatment, such as the removal of both ovaries, which produce hormones. In this case, menopause will begin immediately after the operation, with hormonal changes happening suddenly rather than over a number of years. Doctors used to be more aggressive about removing ovaries for disorders such as endometriosis, says Philadelphia gynecologic surgeon and women's health expert Karen Tang. "They'd say, 'Well, you're forty-nine, your ovaries are quiet anyway, you're not having babies, you're not going to notice the difference.' But now there's been a significant change in the way that we approach surgical menopause."

In the past several years, says Tang, "two major studies showed, with a lot of really great data, that surgical menopause, even into age sixty or more, had much more serious cardiovascular disease and mortality risk, along with things like colon cancer, dementia, and bone thinning. Now we really have to exhaust all other options and have a very good reason to take out the ovaries before we consider doing it. Nowadays, the default is, if you have a hysterectomy, we're not going to touch the ovaries, unless there is an increased risk of ovarian cancer, such as in patients with BRCA mutation, or perhaps in the most severe cases of endometriosis. Because even until you're well into a menopause age range, there are health benefits."

Only the removal of both ovaries brings on automatic menopause, so if you've had a hysterectomy or surgical removal of the uterus, but your ovaries, which make hormones, were *not* removed, your ovaries will continue to put out estrogen until you naturally go through menopause.

The years leading up to menopause, when women may have changes in their monthly cycles, hot flashes, and other symptoms, is called perimenopause. I'm going to talk about perimenopause in detail in chapter 3, but we'll have a preview here.

Perimenopause usually begins in a woman's forties and lasts until menopause, which on average occurs at the age of fifty-one. It may begin as early as thirty-five or as late as fifty-nine. Anything older than forty-five is considered normal, according to Stephanie S. Faubion, medical director of the North American Menopause Society, and about 95 percent of women reach this milestone by age fifty-five.

During perimenopause, the ovaries begin to run out of functioning egg cells and start to close up shop. At the same time, levels of the body's production of estrogen and progesterone, two hormones made by the ovaries that help regulate your menstrual cycle and prepare the body for pregnancy, often begin to fluctuate. As of now, there's no simple test to predict or confirm menopause or perimenopause. (A 2021 Finnish study found, perhaps unsurprisingly, that one telltale indication menopause was imminent was when participants tended to "increase their alcohol consumption.") But an accurate diagnosis can be made by a doctor after hearing your symptoms and medical history.

Once you've gone through a full year without having a period, you've officially reached menopause—and perimenopause is over. If you go eleven months without a period and the Crimson Tide rolls back in, you start over—as I learned at perhaps the worst possible moment.

I was on assignment for *Vogue*, doing a story on open-water swimming—a sport particularly popular in Europe, in which you swim, usually with a group, in open bodies of water such as oceans, lakes, or rivers. It's more demanding than swimming in a pool, thanks to variabilities in waves, wind, currents, and weather, and having to dodge motorboats and jet skiers, but it's still doable for a middling athlete like me. The assignment took place over a week in the Bahamas—okay, yes, a dream assignment, but for every one of these sparkling gems, I do a hundred stories on gastrointestinal disorders or Eight Ways to Deal with Back Pain.

Sometimes when I pitch trend stories to editors, I fail to think things through. This was the case when I was perched on the edge of a boat near Great Exuma Island, peering grimly into the water before I leaped in. Why was I doing this again? I had trained a bit on the ocean and was a decent swimmer, but the water wasn't clear enough to see to the bottom. What was cruising around down there? The Bahamian seas are home to around forty kinds of sharks. "Oh, most of them are harmless," scoffed my guide, an imperturbable South African. "You won't see any, except maybe nurse sharks, and they usually won't bother you."

I tried hard not to fixate on the words *most of them* and *usually*.

I was the last of a dozen people in my group to jump in the water. As we began our long swim, a boat trailing alongside us, I relaxed a little—although I'm not proud to report that I quickly wormed my way into the center of my swimming pod, reasoning that at least I wouldn't be picked off first by predators.

The more practiced swimmers surged ahead, leaving me with one of the instructors. *Okay, this is actually fun,* I thought happily, and did a little dive under the water to scout for life.

Sea creature fun facts: Aside from humans, the one species known to experience menopause are toothed whales—belugas, narwhals, killer whales, and short-finned pilot whales. And it appears that those who have undergone menopause aren't cast aside by cetacean society.

A team of British researchers found that postmenopausal killer whales have the biggest impact on their grand-calves' chance of survival. In an oceanic version of the grandmother hypothesis, it seems the post-reproductive grandmothers "are the most knowledgeable and provide an important leadership role in the group when foraging in salmon grounds." In pods without Grandma's crucial intel of "regions of salmon abundance," more calves died sooner.

But back to my Bahamian adventure. After I scanned the seawater around me, I popped back up, alarmed. "There's a school of silver fish behind us," I gabbled to the guide, pointing. "They're big, *very* big. I . . ."

She smoothly dived under. "Yep, barracuda," she said as she surfaced. "It's actually called a battery of barracuda. I'd say there are about twenty."

"What if they get any closer?" I asked in what I hoped was an offhand way.

"Oh, you just give them a punch in the nose," she said cheerfully. She explained that they're attracted to the flash of jewelry, which mimics the scales of fish, and blood. Otherwise, she added, they usually stay clear.

Again with the *usually*! I had taken off my jewelry and exhibited no sign of blood, I told her. I didn't have any cuts, and I hadn't had my period in almost a year. That ship, I told her, had sailed.

"It happened far too early for me, and I wasn't prepared. It was a shock. I felt very isolated."

–Naomi Watts

"Then you're fine," she said. "They'll follow at a distance." I told myself to keep swimming and ignore the "region of barracuda abundance."

An hour later, one of my fellow swimmers freestyled over to me. "Everything okay?" she asked. "Did you cut yourself?"

I felt around, alarmed. Maybe I brushed up against some coral? I looked down. A vivid ribbon of red trailed out of the end of my bathing suit. As I floated, it grew larger until a red cloud enveloped me. Right outside the cloud, the water flashed silver as the waves began to churn.

Keeping my eyes resolutely forward and willing myself not to scream, I swam with careful, deliberate strokes over to the boat, a crimson plume floating in my wake. *Steady, girl,* I told myself. *Steady.*

I heaved myself onto the deck, still bleeding. One swimmer, an athletic woman in her seventies, followed me up and wrapped me in a towel. As I lay quietly on the deck, the towel soon soaked through with blood. My fellow swimmers told me later that I looked like someone had murdered me and wrapped up my body for disposal.

• • • •

How many of us have formulated any sort of game plan for this significant transition that will, potentially, take up a third of our lives? People who are going to be parents find it helpful to be prepared—reading books, consulting with friends and family, watching how-to videos, buying products.

My menopausal comrades are largely on their own. As there are few medical guidelines on how to handle the menopause transition, let alone social or work support systems, the onus is unfortunately on us to seek the care we need. Women's health experts say that how we manage menopause in midlife will set the stage for our long-term physical and mental health. As your estrogen levels drop, your risk for conditions such as high blood pressure, high cholesterol, and osteoporosis rises. But the more life changes we can make when perimenopause symptoms first appear, the healthier we will be later in life, says Dr. Makeba Williams. "Ideally, I would tell a patient at, say, thirty-seven: 'This is what's coming. Here's how your body may change, how your metabolism might change. These are the potential risks.' Because if I can do this intervention and help her make behavioral and lifestyle and dietary changes, then this life transition will be easier."

Knowledge is power.

Back in Minkin's office, I'm not even finished telling her about my undertaking before she has grabbed a notebook and is busily scribbling a list of doctors, researchers, and colleagues that I should contact. "You should definitely talk to Hadine Joffe about sleep. She's a buddy of mine," she says.

This generous impulse, I will come to find, is typical. In my many years of health reporting, I have never encountered a more supportive, collegial bunch than menopause experts. "We're not the glitz and glamour of the pregnancy stuff or fertility stuff," says Joffe when I duly phone Minkin's "buddy" later. "Nobody is like, 'Rah-rah, put these people front and center!'" She laughs. "My husband says that it seems like everyone has to tell me their menopause story. Well, it affects a big part of the population. It's not some rare thing."

I started this project because I wanted to know this information for myself. But as I dug deeper, I got caught up in these physicians' zeal and passion for their work. *Sound advice on getting through menopause—in relative comfort and in good health—should* not *be this hard to find*, I kept thinking. I was filled with an almost righteous indignation. *I deserve to feel better*, I said to myself. *All of us deserve to feel better!*

Almost every time I talked to a menopause expert, I'd receive a flurry of follow-up emails and recommendations. "Have you contacted Pauline Maki? She's doing really interesting brain research. Oh, be sure to talk to Nanette Santoro about a medication called fezolinetant, it's super-exciting."

These experts obligingly phoned me between clinical appointments, from the lab, on weekends and early mornings before work. Dr. Williams called me as she rushed on her lunch hour to get party supplies for her nine-year-old daughter's birthday. While I was on a Zoom call with Dr. Rubin, the urologist, conducted during the manic hour between her work shift and her kids' bedtime, she asked me if I was considering hormone therapy. I told her I was.

Five minutes after I hung up, she had located two prominent urologists within a thirty-minute drive of my house. *Go talk to these two doctors,* she wrote, and included links.

If these experts had their way, they tell me over and over again, every woman would have a medical team to help her navigate menopause. As this is not the world in which we currently live (women's healthcare is, as Dr. Rubin puts it, "a nightmare at every juncture"), I am going to assemble this team for you. I will interview the best experts in the country, among them ob-gyns, sleep experts, dermatologists, and psychologists.

With their guidance, I will lay out a clear plan of action, along with the latest research and information on treatments and medications. I will provide a script so that you can tell your family and friends about what's going on with your body and mind, without awkwardness or shame. I will investigate hormone therapy, increasingly found to be safer than previously thought. And I will suggest conversation starters for your doctor so you can get the treatment you need.

The days of suffering in silence are over. "What many people don't know is that with interventions, we can help with most things," says Dr. Minkin, handing me a list of experts to contact. She smiles. "My message is, you don't have to be miserable. There are almost no symptoms that we can't make better."

Onward.

· Chapter 3 ·

The Twilight Saga

Why the Hell Didn't Anyone Tell Me About Perimenopause?

I've written for magazines for three decades, and one aspect of the job that still makes me jittery, even with long experience, is interviewing celebrities. Over the years, I've profiled hundreds of famous people. It never gets any easier. When I first started out, in the pre-internet heyday of magazines, I was able to spend days with celebrities. Now I get an hour at most, and sometimes half an hour, for a cover story, so I need to make every second count. If the famous person is in a bad mood, I lose valuable minutes as I attempt to jolly them up.

I prepare by studying everything ever written about my celebrity as if it's ancient sacred text. That way, when I casually drop the name of their second-grade guinea pig, I convey that I have done my homework, they are then reassured, and it becomes slightly more possible that they relax their guard a bit. In my opening chitchat, I talk about them, never about me, which causes celebrity eyes to immediately glaze over. I labor mightily to get them to be at least somewhat receptive toward me. Want to see a notoriously humorless celebrity bloom? Tell them, "Wow, you're hilarious! Why isn't it out there how *funny* you are?" If my subject is in their twenties, I tee up with a question about their astrological sign.

I've sweated through many awkward situations over the years, but my perimenopausal perspiring was about to go to another level.

During the pandemic lockdown, I was given an assignment to interview, over two long Zoom calls, a lovely, personable TV and film star in her early twenties. A few days before our chat, I writhed through a series of scorching hot flashes and night sweats—which lingered into the day, so that after a while they were just "sweats."

The morning of our appointment, I woke up feeling like I had been boiled like a dumpling; it was as if my bedroom ceiling had flooded and drenched me.

Stress has been shown to be a potential trigger for hot flashes—and my keyed-up state was undoubtedly making them worse. I took a shower but was soon wet again. Dripping and wild-eyed, I looked like a walking mug shot. Appearing deranged was not the way to win someone over, and a twenty-two-year-old isn't going to understand the molten intensity of hot flashes.

I set up my computer in a quiet room for the Zoom call, grabbed the two electric fans I keep on hand, and called a neighbor for a third. Then I positioned them strategically: two below my desk on the left and right, and one on the desk, but at the lightest setting. (I didn't want to look like Stevie Nicks in the "Stand Back" video, which would be a distraction.)

One hour to go and rivulets are trickling down my face and neck. I put on waterproof mascara and a bold lip. I have a notebook full of my questions written down—never electronic, which could break or run out of power—I just have to be careful not to drip onto the paper. I'm the melting-face emoji come to life, so I hurry to the bathroom for tissues. Fifteen minutes. Crap, we're out of tissues! I grab a wad of toilet paper and race to the computer. The running, of course, has caused my facial tributaries to feed into a stream.

I tuck the clump of toilet paper into the sleeve of my sweater, just like my grandma once did. That way I can surreptitiously dab my face while pretending to move a strand of hair.

Aaaaaand it's showtime. "Hiiiii," I say with a manic grin. "How has your day been?"

• • • •

Some six thousand women a day enter perimenopause. For the majority, perimenopause is a phase of life that begins when they are in their forties—just for perspective, that's Beyoncé, not *The Golden Girls'* Bea Arthur.

Yet many don't even know it exists. A 2022 survey from Bonafide, a company that makes menopause products, found that nearly a third of the U.S. women surveyed were "not aware" of perimenopause.

However dismaying this might be, it is not a shocker. According to the *Merriam-Webster Collegiate Dictionary*, *perimenopause* first surfaced in the lexicon in 1962, but on Google Books's Ngram Viewer, a search engine that charts word frequencies in books, *perimenopause* isn't mentioned at all until the 1990s. The word didn't appear in *The New York Times* until 1997. As I write this, the word *perimenopause* is flagged by Microsoft Word's spell-check, even though it's spelled correctly. I guess it doesn't yet qualify as a legitimate word (then again, as of 2021, just 29.7 percent of Microsoft's global workforce was female).

In the UK, at least, which is leagues ahead of the United States in terms of menopause awareness both on a policy and a social level, Amazon's cloud-based voice assistant Alexa will now give an answer to the question "What is perimenopause?" (As well as to "What are the risks of hormone replacement therapy for menopause?") American Alexa must feel that it's still a shameful topic.

Even in the medical literature, writes Dr. Nanette Santoro in the *Journal of Women's Health*, perimenopause is an "ill-defined time period that surrounds the final years of a woman's reproductive life." It wasn't until the 1980s, she writes, that longitudinal studies—which follow the same group of women for years—shed some much-needed light on the role of hormones during menopause.

Perimenopause is different for everyone, but for many, it can be a hormonal road that's just as rocky as puberty. Worse, these symptoms often overlap—hot flashes cause sleep loss, which can exacerbate depression, and so on. It's kind of like PMS, only—*wheeeee!*—it's daily.

Irritatingly, perimenopause often occurs right when women are juggling the most responsibilities of their lives. They're running households, sometimes raising children, and often caring for aging parents, too. If they're working outside the home, they're likely just hitting their stride in their career (according to salary site Payscale, women's salaries are highest at age forty-four).

Doctors once believed that menopause was a slow diminishing of estrogen levels, which dwindled year by year until the last menstrual period. Now research has shown that perimenopause—defined by the Johns Hopkins website as the transitional time *before* menopause when your ovaries begin winding down—is not a gradual downshift. Instead, it's often chaotic and disruptive. As levels of estrogen drop further, many women experience a host of menopause-like symptoms, from hot flashes to sleep problems.

Many women in perimenopause also weather a dramatic uptick

"When you get into
perimenopause, you notice
the hormonal changes happening,
the sweating, the moods—you're
just like, all of a sudden, furious
for no reason. I think menopause
gets a really bad rap and needs
a bit of a rebranding. I don't think
we have in our society a great
example of an aspirational
menopausal woman."

—Gwyneth Paltrow

in bleeding, called menorrhagia, like my crime-scene episode on the boat. It soaks through clothes, can last months, and in some cases can leave people housebound. It's not uncommon for women in perimenopause to have prolonged bleeding for ten or more days. Sometimes it's so heavy that they assume they have a terrible injury or a disease and hurry to the emergency room.

My friend Lisa bled profusely for a month straight. "It was so bad, I had to put a garbage bag on the couch in case it leaked through," she says. "I'd wear double pads but still wake up in the night a bunch of times to change my overnight pad." One day she passed out—thankfully, not at the law firm where she's a receptionist, but at home on a weekend. "I thought, *Okay, I can't do this anymore,* and I got a Mirena IUD. That finally stopped it."

In a noteworthy 2022 episode of *And Just Like That . . .* titled "No Strings Attached," the character Charlotte York Goldenblatt, who hadn't gotten her period in four months, assumed she "did not have to deal with this shit anymore" and was finally in menopause. She learned otherwise one afternoon when she met her friends for lunch and was suddenly visited by what Miranda deemed a "flash period," which bloomed darkly on Charlotte's snow-white jumpsuit.

Flash period is not a medical term, but the experience of having your "wacky periods go all over the place" is common, says Dr. Mary Jane Minkin of Yale Medical School. While we think of perimenopause as the lowering of estrogen, in fact many of the miseries of this stage of life are because estrogen can spike unexpectedly, not because it's lacking.

Perimenopause, according to the National Institutes of Health, usually lasts around seven years, but it can drag on as long as fourteen years.

How long it persists depends on a number of factors, from

ethnicity to lifestyle habits such as smoking, which can jump-start menopause, research reveals. Genetics have also been shown to play a part. Much like the timing of puberty, it's common for women to reach menopause at a point similar to when their mothers did—which is why it's helpful to know when it occurred. Other factors are not as influential, such as whether you used hormonal birth control. In fact, a Dutch study found no indication that use of oral contraceptives influences menopausal age (although if you're on the Pill, it may hide or control some of the symptoms of menopause, such as night sweats).

During perimenopause, the levels of estrogen (released before ovulation) and progesterone (released after ovulation) in your body rise and fall. Your periods may get lighter or heavier, shorter or longer. Sometimes they can last a week—as mine did—or even longer, at which point women can lose so much blood that they become anemic and need to take iron supplements.

It may be tempting during this tumultuous time to take some sort of menopause test for confirmation. But because hormone levels change drastically throughout a menstrual cycle during the menopause transition, hormone tests to determine your menopause status, although popular, are usually not helpful, according to the North American Menopause Society's menopause guidebook.

In a typical menstrual cycle, ovaries produce estrogen, which builds up the lining of the uterus, called the endometrium, to allow implantation of an embryo. Halfway through your cycle, you ovulate and a mature follicle carrying an egg is released. If you don't get pregnant, this triggers production of progesterone, which breaks down the endometrium, which then bleeds out in the form of a period—known, charmingly in Germany, as "strawberry week."

As perimenopause occurs and the ovaries function less consistently, estrogen production becomes erratic, we ovulate less well, and we make less progesterone, says Minkin. She and other practitioners use the metaphor of a lawn to explain the relationship between estrogen and progesterone. Picture the endometrium as the grass. Estrogen is the fertilizer that causes the grass to grow. Think of progesterone is the lawn mower that *cuts* the grass. When you make less progesterone, says Minkin, "you end up with overgrowth and funky, erratic bleeding."

Which is also why natural family planning, or the rhythm method, used to disastrous effect by Tom and me in Chapter 1, is not encouraged during perimenopause, because irregular periods make predicting fertile times tough. Also, if you're still bleeding, you're still ovulating. During this time, you can absolutely still get pregnant, like Minkin's patients with later-in-life "surprise" babies, so do not toss the birth control. For healthy women in perimenopause with so-called funky bleeds, Minkin says, "we can just give them progesterone. Low-dose birth control pills can also be a blessing in perimenopause."

Humans, by the way, aren't the only ones who get funky bleeds. While menstruation is rare in mammals, it has long been known that primates and bats have periods. In 2016, researchers at Monash University in Clayton, Australia, were excited to discover yet another species visited by Aunt Flo: the common spiny mouse, the "first known menstruating rodent." They noticed what appeared to be "menstrual-like anomalies" on the vaginas of a colony of spiny mice, which are a mainstay in medical laboratories. To track the mice's periods, the team flushed their tiny vaginas with saline solution daily and analyzed their cells.

The common spiny mouse's menstruation, as it turns out, is almost uncannily like ours. Researchers found that they spend roughly the same percentage of their cycle menstruating as people do, and they even seem to get a form of PMS, during which they eat more, have anxiety, demonstrate an "elevated preference" for isolation, and resist touching (*Get the hell away from me!*).

A later 2021 study found that spiny mice have a gradual, rather than a sudden, transition to menopause—suggesting that they also go through a kind of perimenopause, which makes me feel a kinship to my spiny mouse sisters.

• • • •

If Niagara Falls–like flow is making you miserable, there are several solutions to discuss with your doctor. First, have them rule out other causes for heavy bleeding, such as polyps or fibroids. While you're there, consider whether you need to take a blood test to check your iron levels. Iron-deficiency anemia is common with heavy periods, when you lose a lot of blood and your iron stores are depleted. Without enough iron, your body can't produce enough hemoglobin, a substance in red blood cells that helps carry oxygenated blood throughout your body. If you have iron deficiency anemia, you may feel light-headedness or major fatigue, or you might be short of breath.

An iron supplement can shore up your body's iron supply. Look for gentle iron supplements, which are easier on the stomach, and, crucially, non-constipating.

There are several nonhormonal treatments that you can take when you're bleeding (as opposed to hormonal treatments, which are taken all the time). One is tranexamic acid (Lysteda), an oral medication that's FDA-approved for heavy menstrual bleeding. It prevents the breakdown of a protein called fibrin, the main protein in a blood clot. Studies show it can reduce bleeding by about half, which can be a godsend.

If you'd rather take over-the-counter meds, ibuprofen, surprisingly, has been shown to decrease the deluge by 25 to 30 percent.

Why? It slows down production of a hormone called prostaglandin, which causes uterine contractions that help your body shed the lining of your uterus—aka your menstrual cramps. Less prostaglandin means less uterine shedding means less bleeding. (Also, ibuprofen relieves cramping.)

As for hormonal options, oral contraceptives not only provide birth control but help regulate your menstrual cycle, which can steady the prodigious bleeding.

If you don't want to take daily pills, a hormonal IUD (intrauterine device) that's inserted in your uterus, like my friend's Mirena IUD, releases a type of progesterone that keeps the lining of your uterus thin and cuts down on the bleeding. Depending on the brand, it doesn't have to be replaced for three to seven years, either, so you can set it and forget it.

For the perimenopausal woman who is a mother, home can be an unceasing hormonal tsunami if she has a teenage daughter who is going through puberty at the same time. All parties may be dealing with odd BO, morphing body shapes, and seesawing moods. In a song called "Hormones" that describes this dynamic, Tracey Thorn sings, "You're stampin' up the stairs, I'm cryin' at the kitchen sink."

This overlap of perimenopause and puberty may be getting more common as the age of first-time moms continues to creep upward. The average age in the United States of a first-time mother, according to the CDC, is now twenty-six, up from twenty-two in 1975. If perimenopause starts in the mid-forties, then more and more mothers are entering a major identity shift at the same time as their kids.

My friend Thea started going through perimenopause when her two daughters became teenagers. "There's a lot of door-slamming," she says. "And none of us are sleeping. I have hot flashes and night sweats, and they're up late, even though I yell at them to go to bed, so all of us are sleep-deprived." (Thea's yelling may not help: research shows that after puberty, a teen's circadian rhythms typically shift about two hours later, a change known as a sleep phase delay.)

"My girls both push me away, but they still need me, too, while I just want to be alone," Thea goes on. "I think the main difference between me and them is that I remember what it was like to be a teen and how painful it could be, so I give them some slack. They just think I'm losing my shit for no reason."

I may have a similar situation going on in my house with my own teenage daughter, but given that the list of things I do that mortifies her is already lengthy—including chewing cereal "weirdly," wearing sweatpants that are "sad," and, the worst sin, speaking directly to her friends as I'm driving them around—I should probably avoid writing about this.

• • • •

As financier Bernard M. Baruch aptly put it, "To me, old age is fifteen years older than I am." When your life is teeming with responsibilities and you're trying to make it to the finish line every day, perimenopause and menopause are easy issues to put aside. Don't do it, says Dr. Makeba Williams. She starts talking to patients about perimenopause while they're in their forties, sometimes even in their thirties. The sooner you can identify your symptoms, she says, the earlier you can manage them.

If you're noticing some changes that seem like perimenopause, here are some ways to get ahead of it.

If you're in your forties, **be mindful of what experts call the "core four" perimenopausal symptoms that tend to appear along with those funky bleeds**: hot flashes, crappy sleep, vaginal dryness, and depression. The minute you begin to discern a pattern, take

"Perimenopause and menopause should be treated as the rites of passage that they are. How wonderful would it be if we could get to a place where we are able to have these conversations openly and without shame—and admit, freely, that this is what's going on, so we don't feel like we're going insane?"

—Gillian Anderson

notes for your doctor. I'm going to talk about each of these symptoms in turn in the chapters that follow.

"Brain fog" can also take hold in perimenopause. Studies show estrogen is neuroprotective, meaning that it protects neurons in the brain from degeneration. With the arrival of perimenopause, your head can feel like an Etch A Sketch that someone has just given a vigorous shake. (On a happier note, research I'll get into later shows that this fuzziness tends to clear up by menopause. Tiny victories!) "Emotional sensitivity to psychosocial stress" ramps up as well, according to a study from the University of North Carolina at Chapel Hill, thanks to fluctuations in estradiol, a form of estrogen. It results in spikes of anger, irritability, and heightened feelings of rejection in social situations.

During perimenopause, my moods, usually fairly stable, vacillated from manic highs to bouts of sobbing over Serena Williams's Instagram post that her dog Jackie had died. ("I feel so lucky to have such a special friend. Give your dog, cat, pet a big hug. #breakingheart #bff.")

Women are more vulnerable to depression in general—they're nearly twice as likely to be diagnosed with depression as men. A 2021 study in the journal *Psychoneuroendocrinology* finds that perimenopausal depression is often presented as irritability. This was the case with me, too: anything set me off. A locked computer password could incite unleash-the-dragons rage.

If a person has underlying low-level depression, perimenopause can make it worse. Even if a woman does *not* have depression, research shows it's twice as likely to turn up when perimenopause begins. If you find that feelings of grief, anger, or helplessness around perimenopause are getting in the way of daily life, see a mental health professional. Perimenopausal depression has always been underrecognized, but clinical guidelines were finally published in 2018, so at last it might be easier for a doctor to spot.

* * * *

Once you've toted up your symptoms, **talk to a doctor you trust—one who makes you feel heard and understood.** While you may love your ob-gyn or primary care doctor, she may not have the menopause training you need, says Denise Pines, founder of Wise-Pause Wellness, an inclusive menopause community of practitioners. She frequently tells women that if this is the case, consider moving on from your longtime ob-gyn. "Women feel like they can't leave the ob-gyn who delivered their babies, even though their babies are now nineteen or twenty," she says with a laugh. "And they're suffering because their doctors don't have strategies for them. It's okay to see someone else."

Minkin suggests asking your practitioner, "I think I'm in perimenopause, and I understand that going through menopause puts me at greater risk for osteoporosis and cardiovascular disease. Can you tell me how to protect myself?" If you receive a solid, detailed answer, proceed. If not, it's fine to find another doctor. Don't cram all your perimenopause questions into your annual exam, either. The average doctor's visit lasts eighteen minutes, according to a 2021 study published in the journal *Medical Care.* Instead, **make a separate appointment**, says Williams, joining the chorus of many other experts. "You might spend half your life in menopause, and it's really important to give this time period the attention it deserves," she says.

Schedule a consultation along with a complete medical exam. If you're not quite certain that perimenopause is causing your symptoms, it may be tempting to get one of the many tests that have flooded the market that claim they can tell you where you are in your menopause transition by analyzing the hormone levels in your blood, urine, or saliva. Over-the-counter tests usually measure follicle-stimulating hormone (FSH), which is made by your pituitary gland and is important for sexual development. FSH tends to increase in blood levels as a woman approaches menopause.

Save your money, asserts the North American Menopause Society. When it comes to salivary and urine hormone tests, NAMS's position on its website is pretty straightforward. These tests are "expensive, not accurate, and should not be used to evaluate or treat menopause symptoms." They're generally not helpful, contends NAMS, because hormone levels change throughout the menstrual cycle. To date, it concludes, there is no simple test to predict or confirm perimenopause. Instead, as mentioned, your doctor can usually do it by reviewing your medical history and your signs and symptoms.

A helpful way to figure out if menopause is on the horizon, as Dr. Nanette Santoro told *The Washington Post*, is this: if you're over forty-five and have gone sixty days without a period and you used to cycle normally, she says, you've got a 90 percent chance of being menopausal within four years.

If you're not getting anywhere with your doctor, another option beyond switching physicians is to **see a menopause specialist** for an individualized treatment plan—which is critically important, as every woman experiences this life stage differently. (There's no "one" menopause.) Perimenopause isn't like other conditions, where treatment protocols are clear, and a menopause specialist has received additional training on how to navigate this unique life stage. Often, they are ob-gyns—most of the ob-gyns I interview in this book are also certified menopause practitioners—but they can also be, for example, nurse practitioners or naturopathic practitioners.

NAMS's website, Menopause.org, features a long list of certified menopause practitioners who are specifically trained in menopause and midlife healthcare issues. They have met the exacting standards NAMS has set, and must recertify every three years. Simply plug in your zip code to find a certified menopause practitioner near you.

If you don't find a practitioner nearby, says ob-gyn Kameelah Phillips, founder of Calla Women's Health in New York City and a NAMS-certified menopause practitioner herself, "some offer virtual visits, so you can do consults from all over the country," she says. "You may only need to see them once or twice, and sometimes they're less expensive than an office visit."

Given the disparities in menopausal care among ethnic groups—a 2022 study in the journal *Menopause* found that menopausal white women were more likely to be prescribed hormone therapy than Black or Hispanic women, for instance—it's not exactly a shock that some women of color are mistrustful of the medical community. A Penn Medicine analysis of more than one hundred thousand patient surveys found that patients who shared the same ethnic background as their doctor were likely to rate their experience much higher.

"I do think it can be helpful to find a doctor in your community who looks like you," says Phillips. "With that comes a level of trust and honesty that might not immediately be achieved in other circumstances." She thinks for a minute. "But that's tricky, because then it's, 'Oh, she'll see a Black doctor. That's not my responsibility.' When *all* doctors need to step their game up and create an equitable and safe space for everyone."

Denise Pines adds that the media should center stories about menopause around women of color, too, which can empower them to self-advocate. "Because typically when you hear these conversations, they're from one perspective," she says.

When you do find a doctor that you trust, **arrive prepared**. Bring a list of detailed perimenopause symptoms (if you're having hot flashes, for instance, count how many you're having per day, and how long they are) as well as a list of the meds you're taking and a synopsis of both your medical history and your family's medical history. Ask your mom, sisters, and aunts when they went through menopause and let the doctor know. Often doctors helpfully provide forms for your health history online so you can fill them out ahead of time.

Sometimes it can take some sleuthing to pinpoint when your older relatives went through menopause, at a time when women didn't talk about it, even to themselves. "I started getting hot flashes when I was maybe forty," says Mom one afternoon when I swing by her house after receiving a text saying *I've just made a peach cobbler, come over!* "But it's not like I said to myself, *Oh, this must be perimenopause.* Hell, I've never even heard of perimenopause until you told me about it."

"Remember you told me your doctor put you on Premarin when you reached menopause?" I say. "The guy with the cold hands? When was that?"

She shrugs. "Maybe my late forties? Who can remember?"

I keep pressing. "Do you remember any life events at that time? Who was president? Was it Reagan?"

"No idea," she says. "Let's say forty-eight?"

Even if you can get only ballpark numbers like my mother provided, they are useful for more than just an indication of when you may go through menopause yourself. If you are in your late thirties and are getting irregular periods, but your female relatives didn't hit menopause until they were, say, in their fifties, that is the sort of red flag that is good for a doctor to know about.

As mentioned earlier, heavy bleeding can also be a sign of conditions like polyps, cysts, certain cancers, and fibroids. Three or more missed periods in women younger than forty might indicate primary ovarian insufficiency (POI), among other causes. During this critical time period, there are so many things that a physician can catch. Some symptoms of hyperthyroidism, when the thyroid gland produces too much thyroid hormone, can mimic the menopause transition, with symptoms such as hot flashes and heart palpitations.

Assemble your family history of cancer, breast cancer, and gynecologic cancer, including how old your relatives were when it happened and how they were treated. Bring any history of bone health, too. Did your mother or grandma ever fracture a hip, and if so, how old were they? If any were under sixty-five, which is less common, this is worth noting. (If you have a history of osteoporosis in your family, your insurance should pay for a DEXA scan, a painless bone density test that will assess the strength of your bones.)

Provide your family history of any cardiovascular disease as well, because this is still the leading cause of death for women. As your body loses estrogen, you lose its protective effects on your heart (something I'll discuss in later chapters). In 2020, the American Heart Association released a statement that some of the symptoms common with menopause have a correlation with cardiovascular disease—among them hot flashes, night sweats, depression, sleep disturbances, and increased abdominal fat—so heart health, it went on, should be monitored in midlife.

With your physicians, **formulate a game plan** for your menopause transition. Menopause signals a time, says Anna Camille Moreno, DO, a menopause practitioner at Duke University Medical Center, when you could be at higher risk for hypertension, cholesterol disorders, osteoporosis, and diabetes. As doctors love to say, preventive care is vastly preferable to reactive care. Perimenopause, say many experts, is the ideal time to get your shit together, health-wise. The good news is that effective treatments abound—yet many women have no idea these exist. I'll delve into them in later chapters, but here are a few examples.

For perimenopausal hot flashes, **estrogen-based therapies** are the most effective choice. (I'll do a deep dive into hormones in chapter 9.) If you're leery of hormones, a solid nonhormonal option is the FDA-approved Brisdelle, a selective serotonin reuptake inhibitor (SSRI). For women who have hot flashes that are disruptive only at night, a 2020 meta-analysis of the antiseizure medication gabapentin found that it was very beneficial. For vaginal dryness, ospemiphine (brand name Osphena) is a daily nonhormonal pill that fortifies cells in fragile vaginal tissue.

One crucial area of premenopause preparation, finds researchers at the University of Copenhagen, is **to be as physically active as possible**, when estrogen levels are high—in order to form, and bank, as many capillaries in your muscles as you can. Not-so-fun fact: After menopause, you can still build muscle, but you can't form new capillaries. The more capillaries you have as you enter menopause, they found, the more robust your muscles *after* menopause. Given that the number of over-forty women who have entered U.S. triathlons has recently doubled, this is helpful news.

This is a good time to **keep an eye on your weight**, too. A 2022 study published in the journal *Menopause* found that the greatest increases in the overall percentage of body fat and decreases in lean muscle mass occur during perimenopause—which, they say, may be the most "optimal intervention window" to make lifestyle changes. By the time women get to menopause—which, again, begins at about the age of fifty-one for many—they found that it's both harder for the body to use fat for fuel and it has an increased resistance to muscle building.

Diet is just as important. The Mediterranean diet—the regimen that's heavy on plants, whole grains, olive oil, and fish that is beloved by physicians—has been found to be "comparable with pharmacological interventions in terms of reducing the risk of cardiovascular events" among menopausal women, according to a 2020 report published in the journal *Critical Reviews in Food Science and Nutrition*. This is no small thing. In addition, investigators at the University of Leeds who tracked more than 14,000 British women for four years found that natural menopause arrived one to three years later among those who ate a lot of legumes and oily fish.

Women can lose up to 20 percent of their bone density during the menopause transition due to waning estrogen levels, according to the Endocrine Society, so **be sure to get the recommended daily allowance of calcium**, which keeps bones dense and strong. The National Institutes of Health recommend 1,200 milligrams of calcium a day for women ages thirteen through seventy—ideally through food, says Dr. Anna Camille Moreno. Moreno has patients use an online calcium calculator, like the one from the National Osteoporosis Foundation. "They plug in what they're eating every day, see how much calcium they're getting, and then the calculator tells them what they should take in a calcium supplement to make up the difference," she says. Eat a six-ounce container of yogurt, and you're a quarter of the way there. (Greek yogurt may have a better reputation than regular yogurt, but a little-known fact is that it loses some of its calcium during the straining process.) The National Institutes of Health also recommend 600 IU of vitamin D for women ages fifty to seventy, which helps your body absorb calcium. "Vitamin D_3 is a big part of bone health," says Moreno, who usually has patients take 1,000 to 2,000 IUs daily. "It doesn't reverse bone loss, but it really helps the interconnections of those bones."

Here's a sobering fact: the Bone Health & Osteoporosis Foundation maintains that one in *two* women over fifty will break a bone because of osteoporosis.

Perimenopause may also be the time to **take a fresh look at your relationship with alcohol**—which, says Williams, contributes to weight gain, can interfere with sleep, and can be a trigger for hot flashes. Moderate drinking for women—defined by the U.S. Dietary Guidelines as one drink a day—is associated with a lower risk of heart disease and dementia. Two and up, however, may harm a woman's health, according to the North American Menopause Society. Yet a 2020 SWAN study of alcohol use among women across the menopausal transition found that women were "more likely to transition from non-excessive to excessive drinking" during the early perimenopausal stage.

Perimenopause is an ideal time to **step away from the cigarettes.** Smoking has been shown, in a study of 79,000 women published in the journal *Tobacco Control*, to bring on menopause by a not-insignificant twenty-one months. That means less time with the protective benefits of estrogen on bones, brain, and heart.

Have more sex, and you can perhaps delay menopause even further. Women who have sex weekly, or even monthly, according to researchers at University College London, have a lower risk of entering menopause early, compared to those who report having some form of sex less than monthly. (That includes self-stimulation, so a partner isn't necessary.)

Overall: **Think of perimenopause as the perfect time to assess and reset**, says Williams. "We should not be looking at this as a time of, like, 'My ovaries have failed, I have no more reproductive potential, and therefore I don't have any potential in life. I might as well close up shop and just wait for death,'" she says. (Mordant humor is another characteristic that menopause experts seem to share.)

Instead, she says, we should be figuring out how to fully optimize our health for the next half of our lives.

• • • •

Perimenopause is more than a collection of symptoms. It can completely upend your identity. When you're in your forties—what some might deem life's very prime—your self-image may be that of a striving professional, a young(ish) mother, an athlete.

After my doctor told me that I had begun menopause, I was confronted with my own internalized ageism as various negative images arose in my brain: liver spots spattered on a hand reaching for a jar of Centrum Silver, the specter of a closet full of nothing but roomy Eileen Fisher tunics. ("Eileen Fisher" or "Chico's" has become snarky shorthand in some circles for "a woman of a certain age.") I cringe as I recall the sneering, ageist jokes that my stupid teenage friends and I used to make about our middle-aged moms.

When I worked as a staff writer for *Rolling Stone* in my twenties, I regularly interviewed some of the most famous women in music. If any happened to be over fifty, I was inevitably instructed by the editors to ask how they "felt" about aging. At the time, I was blithely unaware of how incredibly annoying that unrelenting question is—especially coming from a twenty-five-year-old. And many of the women I interviewed had already made their opinions known, anyway (like Cher, who once tweeted that "being older than Methuselah Sucks The Big 1").

Maybe I made snide jokes to distance myself from my awareness of my own mortality. Perimenopause can bring up some of your most atavistic fears. Like those barracudas trailing me in the open ocean, a host of deeper issues flit below the surface—anxieties about your waning vitality, attractiveness, and social relevance; fear of invisibility; the gradual loss of power of your body and mind.

Melissa Robinson-Brown, a clinical psychologist in New York City and an assistant clinical professor of psychiatry at Mount Sinai, says that perimenopause can unleash a typhoon of emotions for women (she thoughtfully uses the term *female-born individuals*). They can feel sorrow when they realize that they can't have children anymore, she says, even if they had made a decision not too long ago. "Logically, we know that having children is not the defining moment of womanhood, but some female-born individuals do feel grief that that window is now closing," says Robinson-Brown. "Because it is a loss. They are, in a sense, being forced to retire."

It's also common, she adds, to feel anxiety about how menopause is going to impact your body, and fear concerning how you are going to be perceived by others. "But these are thoughts, and we have the power to shift them." There's a concept called *internal locus of control,* says Robinson-Brown, "which means what happens to us is in our hands. If we adopt an external locus of control, that means our happiness is defined by others. It's so important to not allow anyone else to define you other than yourself. We have a choice regarding what to believe."

Robinson-Brown says to treat this passage as a milestone. "Milestones warrant celebration, and even a change to reflect a new phase in your life," she says. "Don't like your hair? Head to the salon and make a change. Take a healthy risk and go ahead and get that short cut and dye it purple. You know you want to." (The last time I saw Dr. Robinson-Brown, she happened to have short purple hair.)

All transitions, she says, come with a possibility for positive change. "Reflecting on what's lost is a part of the process, but it's also just as important to turn to what's gained. If you have kids, they may be older, meaning more free time for you. You may be more advanced in your career, or beginning a new one, which can also be exciting. It's a time to potentially travel, start new hobbies, go out more, reconnect with old friends."

One way I started coping is through humor. While I've always scrupulously avoided making self-effacing remarks about my face or body, I began to trade joking texts with perimenopausal friends. *When you look down at your phone and see your reflection*, I wrote, *which historical figure do you resemble?* Mine was the magnificently jowled John Quincy Adams, complete with white chin hairs.

The responses rolled in: *Johann Sebastian Bach. Mahatma Gandhi.* Mostly I find these jokes comforting because we share the same lived experience, but sometimes they make me feel dispirited.

"We are always the same age inside," Gertrude Stein once remarked. This resonates with me; my almost-demonically energetic mother and I have agreed that inside, we both feel about thirty. "Sometimes twenty-five on a really good day," says Mom.

• Chapter 4 •

Your Smokin' Hot New Body

Hot Flashes Are More Than a "Nuisance"

I love women who are in midlife; they do not screw around. They no longer squander their time, as they may have done in, say, their twenties. They have had the realization that life is finite, and thus tend to get directly to the point.

Not long ago, I fell into a deep conversation at a barbecue with a woman in her fifties whom I had just met. Within a minute, she told me her dad had recently died, and tears suddenly spilled down her cheeks. I guided her over to a couch, sat her down, and asked her to tell me all about him. She wept while I held her hand and listened.

"People are staring at us," she whispered through tears.

"Who gives a crap," I whispered back.

I find, over and over, that women in midlife have a surplus of empathy as well, having weathered some knocks, like my new friend at the barbecue. (This is the age when, as my mother sagely observes, "shit starts to happen.") Adept at keeping a thousand plates spinning at once, they know how to do things quickly and efficiently, with minimum fuss. If you're in a group of women who are squarely in midlife and one pipes up and announces that she has a problem, someone in that group is going to find a solution.

That is the case one afternoon in my living room as I sit on a couch, nervously petting my snaggle-toothed rescue cat, who is dozing woozily in my lap. Am I really about to discuss my hormonal havoc—my vaginal dryness and weird new thinning hair—with a dozen strangers?

Apparently I am. I'm attending a virtual meeting of the Menopause Café, a pop-up café established in the UK, in which people, usually strangers, gather for liberatingly frank chats. For one day, a café is transformed into a space where they can meet up, have tea and cake, talk confidentially about what they're going through, trade tips, and offer support.

I tense up as a dozen faces appear on-screen. But after a few awkward minutes, the conversation begins to flow. Soon we are discussing not only our hot flashes but painful vaginal dryness in delightfully granular detail. Although I have rarely talked about my symptoms, even with friends, it's easier to do, somehow, with these kindly strangers.

The event's simple guidelines—respect everyone's privacy, no pushing any specific products or services, extend a warm welcome to all genders and ages—were established by Rachel Weiss, who runs her own counseling consultancy in Perth, Scotland.

Weiss got the idea for a Menopause Café after she ran a Death Café, in which strangers meet to have a free-flowing conversation about the mother of all taboo subjects; it occurred to her that menopause was a topic that was similarly off-limits. She asked Death Café founder Jon Underwood if she could set up a Menopause Café using the model he had established, and he readily agreed.

In June of 2017, Weiss, her husband, Andy, and two friends secured a café in Perth called the Blend Coffee Lounge, a homey place with yellow walls and squishy leather sofas. Then they set up a website. *Come join us to drink tea, eat cake, and talk menopause in a safe, confidential environment*, read the first post.

The night of the event, the little group of four sat at a table, nervously eyeing the door. Two baristas waited at the counter. Carrot cake, coffee cake, and scones were arrayed on trays. Would anyone turn up? Was it possible menopause was a subject more taboo than . . . dying? Were they going to have to eat all the carrot cake themselves?

Then people started filtering in. "Oh, god, we were so relieved," recalls Weiss.

She had everyone sit in groups at small tables. To encourage mixing, she told participants if they felt they had nothing to contribute, they could simply get up and go to another table. "That didn't happen," she said with a laugh. "The feedback form said, 'We're British. We feel rude just getting up from the table. Please ring a bell every twenty minutes.'" This method has been used ever since.

The participants swapped advice, but also tackled larger issues, such as: Is now the time to think about "I want" or "I need" rather than "I must" or "I should"? Is my changing body forcing me to put myself first after decades of putting others first, whether through family or work?

The guidelines Weiss had set up worked well, "although in that first meeting, one woman did go on about magnetic knickers," she recalls.

Allow me to explain: menopause magnets, designed to be attached to your underwear, allegedly ease symptoms such as hot flashes by "rebalancing" the sympathetic nervous system by altering your bioenergetic field. Although enthusiastically endorsed by, among others, the Go-Go's singer Belinda Carlisle, who claimed they stopped her relentless hot flashes, there is no scientific evidence that they work.

After the café's successful debut, Weiss was barraged with requests to host another. Soon the Menopause Café spread throughout the UK and then to a dozen other countries, including India (which made national news), Nairobi, and the United States (although there is just one, as of this writing, in Connecticut).

Many cafés take place in person, but some, like the one I attended, are held online. "For some women, there aren't any available in their country, and others are hesitant to enter a room full of strangers," says Weiss.

Weiss dreams of "world domination," with menopause cafés in every country. "I can't tell you how often I've heard 'Now I know I'm not alone' and 'Now I know I'm not going mad,'" she says. "It's just enabling people to have conversations. Taboos keep people silent, which disempowers them." If you're able to chat about the M word more freely, Weiss believes, it's easier to go back to your twenty-eight-year-old male manager and say, "Yes, I really do need a fan at my desk."

• • • •

If people can name anything about menopause at all, they usually bring up hot flashes. Type "menopause" on the stock photo site Shutterstock, and the first image that pops up is the sort of prosperous-looking white lady with a neat gray bob found in ads for high-end cruises as she drinks champagne on deck with her silver-fox husband. She has one hand thrown over her eyes, while the other waves a red fan to cool her hot flashes. The title of the photo, sounding a bit like it was translated into English, is "tired overheated middle-aged lady." There are many of these photos of white ladies wielding various fans, both analog and electric, while only a few photos of gals who have embraced their fate, such as the "happy attractive senior woman in flower field." (At least there's no description of "woman with senile ovaries.")

Hot flashes, menopause's best-known and least-loved signpost, plague up to 80 percent of women. Also known as vasomotor symptoms, they tend, most often, to scorch the face, neck, and chest. Each flash typically lasts between one and five minutes. (Although Dr. Nanette Santoro writes in the *Journal of Women's Health* that "while most women will have an experience of hot flashes limited to just a year or two, others will experience them for a decade or more, *and a small proportion of women will never be free of them* [italics mine]."

Hot flashes can be accompanied by rapid heartbeat, anxiety, and sweating. They range from a sudden, mildly warmish sensation to feeling like you're roasting in front of Satan's space heater.

Hot flashes that occur during sleep are often accompanied by night sweats. When women have these events at night, they get woken up 75 percent of the time, says Dr. Pauline Maki at the University of Illinois at Chicago. "So that means that night after night, week after week, month after month, year after year, women are having a unique type of sleep disturbance related to the fact that they're being woken up because of these thermoregulatory events."

Hot flashes are triggered by hormonal changes, but scientists still don't know exactly how that happens. Research suggests that they occur when plunging estrogen levels cause your body's thermostat (regulated by a gland in your brain called the hypothalamus) to

"The hot flashes are the worst. Sometimes, I feel like I'm going to pass out. They're awful. There's no way in the world men would put up with hot flashes. I think if men had two hot flashes, they would blow the sun up."

–Wanda Sykes

become more sensitive to changes in temperature. When it senses that a woman is too warm, it fires up a hot flash to cool her down, directing blood to vessels in the skin's surface, which then dilate to release body heat and sweat.

The hormonal mayhem that causes your brain's internal thermostat to become more sensitive can also go in the opposite direction and cause *cold* flashes. Cold flashes, less common than hot flashes, can feel like a sudden Arctic blast—made even more frigid if you're sodden from night sweats—and usually pass after a few weird minutes.

Hot flashes can be startlingly intense; in fact, when blood rushes to the vessels nearest the skin, skin temperature may jump seven degrees. I now recognize when friends are on the cusp of a Category 4 hot flash: they stop abruptly in mid-conversation, mutter *Oh hell no*, and look quickly around for an exit in case they need to flee to a quiet place to wait it out. Some women experience heart palpitations so severe that they check into the emergency room; others have what are called tactile hallucinations in which they feel like their skin is *moving*. In severe cases, women can be blasted, like a rotisserie chicken, twenty times daily. A woman in one of Dr. Maki's studies experienced fifty-two flashes in a single day.

One of the many frustrating elements of hot flashes, says Rebecca Thurston, professor of psychiatry, clinical and translational science, epidemiology, and psychology at the University of Pittsburgh, is the surprise. "They come on abruptly throughout the day and the night," she says, "oftentimes without clear contextual cues or triggers."

Originally, conventional wisdom dictated that hot flashes lasted a couple of years at most. "We know now that moderate to severe ones last on average for about seven to ten years," says Thurston. A

2018 Mayo Clinic study found that for some women, hot flashes were persisting into their sixties, seventies, and eighties.

I've been a member of the flash mob three years now; maybe I'll have them until I'm in my eighties, too. As I write this, I had four particularly searing bouts the previous evening, causing me to lurch awake and kick off my covers. I've been trying hard to find an upside to feeling like you're going to spontaneously combust. The only thing I can come up with is that this past winter, we turned off our heat completely at night—my husband would sleep in an igloo if he could—and were able to save a couple of bucks on our heating bill.

As mentioned in chapter 3, when it comes to hot flashes, the disparities among ethnic groups are notable. A 2015 SWAN study found that women of Chinese and Japanese descent in that same study had the shortest duration of hot flashes (experiencing them off and on for 5.4 years and 4.8 years, respectively), while Latinas reported flashes over an average of 8.9 years. Black women had the longest duration of hot flashes, at 10.1 years on average.

Hot flashes aren't the only symptoms shown to impact Black women more during the menopause transition: a 2022 SWAN review of a quarter century of research found that Black women reach menopause eight and a half months earlier than white women and have worse sleep disturbances and depression, but are *less* likely to receive hormone therapy. These disparities, the authors suggested, may have roots in systemic racism. The Black participants in SWAN, they wrote, were born between 1944 and 1954, "and thus grew up in a U.S. society shaped by structural, or institutional, racism embodied in Jim Crow laws." They hypothesized that "structural racism, or 'differential access to the goods, services, and opportunities of society by race,' is a major contributor to health disparities in the cohort."

• • • •

Hot flashes should not be ignored.

For many women, they're more than a mere nuisance. Sleep disruptions caused by hot flashes, for starters, can wreak havoc on mood and metabolism. More significantly, Rebecca Thurston's SWAN research has found that women who experience frequent or persistent hot flashes may be more likely than women who don't get them to experience a heart attack, stroke, or other serious cardiovascular problem years down the line.

These results, Thurston tells me, held true even when traditional cardiovascular risk factors, like smoking, obesity, diabetes, and high blood pressure, were ruled out. It appears that frequent hot flashes are associated with increased blood pressure and higher LDL, or "bad" cholesterol, over time, which can damage the heart and blood vessels.

Heart attacks are the number one cause of death among women (no, it's not breast cancer, as many people mistakenly assume), so this is worth noting. "Look, the last thing that we want to do is scare people," says Thurston. "What I do tell women who have hot flashes is first of all, be on top of your cardiovascular disease risk factors."

Every time you have a hot flash, says Lauren Streicher, a clinical professor of obstetrics and gynecology at Northwestern University's Medical School and medical director of the Northwestern Medicine Center for Sexual Medicine and Menopause, you increase your levels of cortisol, known as the "stress hormone."

"And we know that this impact of the hot flash, the increase in cortisol levels and the inflammatory response, is what is causing women to have this acceleration in heart disease and osteoporosis—all of these other conditions that we know are at higher levels in women who have this inflammatory response," says Streicher. "To me, *this* is the message—that, hello, hot flashes are not something you just tough out. Instead of using all these cooling things that are available, like dressing in layers, so they don't bother you as much, my whole mantra is to eliminate the hot flash."

The most effective treatment to tamp them down is hormone therapy, says Dr. Wen Shen, echoing the opinion of many others. "It really is the gold standard," says Shen.

Menopausal hormone therapy (MHT) involves taking supplemental estrogen daily, in the form of pills, patches, creams, rings, gels, or implants. If you have a uterus, you'll likely need to take progesterone as well, to mitigate the risk of uterine cancer.

Why? Remember that analogy from chapter 3, in which progesterone is the lawn mower that keeps the endometrium "grass" under control? When you're in menopause, you cease shedding your endometrium, the lining of the uterus, by having a period. When the endometrium is no longer shed, estrogen can cause an overgrowth of cells in your uterus, a condition that can lead to cancer. Progesterone reduces the risk of uterine cancer by making the endometrium thin and keeping the overgrowth in check.

In chapter 9, I'll get into the controversy swirling around menopausal hormone therapy, as well as the possible dangers, which vary depending on your age, medical history, and type of treatment. But recent research has found that menopausal hormone therapy prescribed before the age of sixty is more beneficial than risky. Organizations such as NAMS, the Endocrine Society, and the American Society for Reproductive Medicine all share the position that MHT is appropriate for relief of hot flashes for most healthy women who are recently menopausal. ("balance" is a free app that can help you figure out your risk profile.)

"I totally understand the contraindications and that there is a small percentage of women who can't do it, but for the remaining I say, go for it," says an MHT enthusiast named Dianne. She lists her pre-MHT symptoms. "I was angry, super aggressive, sad, completely irrational, with hot flashes so bad I could kill, and had heart palpitations," she says. "But the worst was that I had tired, achy legs, with this dull pain that never went away. I would do 10,000 steps a day, but nothing would ease it." Her doctor put her on MHT, and she started feeling better within weeks. "It took a few adjustments, but it's been six months and I'm a changed woman," she says. "All of those symptoms are gone. I have a new lease on life. Every woman needs access to MHT. I am so frustrated by the way in which the world has thrown the baby out with the water, based on very old, misunderstood research."

If you're leery of hormones or your risk factors make MHT a no-go, several options are available. Know that all have side effects that may be deal-breakers, from constipation to plummeting libido, so hash it out with your doctor.

As mentioned earlier, the only nonhormonal medication approved by the FDA to treat hot flashes is **paroxetine** (Brisdelle), an antidepressant called a selective serotonin reuptake inhibitor (SSRI) that increases serotonin levels in the brain. According to a 2014 study published in the journal *Menopause,* the normal dosage to treat hot flashes is much lower at 7.5 milligrams than what's prescribed for, say, depression (20 to 40 milligrams), which means a lesser chance of the side effects common to higher doses, such as weight gain.

Another antidepressant that physicians use off-label is **venlafaxine** (Effexor), a serotonin and norepinephrine reuptake inhibitor (SNRI) that has also been shown to ease hot flashes. "Venlafaxine is probably the one that people tend to prescribe the most, and it works," says Minkin.

The term *off-label,* by the way, seems somehow illicit, but it simply means that doctors prescribe a drug for a different purpose or condition than what was approved by the FDA. It's called off-label because the medication is being used in a way not described on its package insert. The practice is very common, and it's legal (although know that some insurers will give you a hard time about reimbursement for medications that aren't FDA-approved for the treatment you're getting).

Two promising new hot flash treatments are also on the horizon. **MLE4910**, a compound known as a neurokinin 3 receptor (NK3R) antagonist, was originally developed as a drug for schizophrenia. It was sitting on a shelf, unused, before Waljit Dhillo, a professor of endocrinology and metabolism at Imperial College London, and his team found a new use for it. In the study that Dhillo led, participants felt beneficial effects very quickly—as in a mind-blowing three days—and were able to get rid of nearly three-quarters of their hot flashes in four weeks. The futuristic-sounding MLE4910, says Dhillo, is "game-changing because it's not only highly effective, it can be used by women who can't take hormone therapy." The pharmaceutical company Bayer has already bought a compound, he says, which they'll be developing. Get on it, Bayer!

Another nonhormonal drug in development, called **fezolinetant**, is shaping up to be, as Minkin puts it, "a blockbuster for the hot flash crap." It's a daily oral medication that's known as a receptor blocker, which counteracts the effects of depleted estrogen on the hypothalamus (again, a region of the brain that regulates core body temperature). The FDA has already approved it for treatment of hot flashes, and if all goes well, it should be on the market within a few years. A 2020 study led by Dr. Santoro and published in the journal *Menopause* caused ripples of excitement with the finding that more than half of the women taking fezolinetant in the study reported a reduction of symptoms of a full 90 percent or greater. It didn't take long to start working, either: subjects felt improvements in as early as one week.

Fezolinetant "is on the order of estrogen in its effectiveness, and that just is not true of any of the other non-estrogen alternatives," says Santoro. Some studies, she adds, "have noted an improvement in sleep, too, which would be huge." For women who aren't candidates for hormones or don't wish to take them, "an effective alternative is really a godsend," says Santoro. "About 5 percent of women have hot flashes that never go away, and as they approach their seventies, hormones are not a good choice for them because they carry more risk."

Maki, among others, is both excited by fezolinetant's potential and apprehensive that it will prompt women to bypass hormone therapy entirely. "I'm concerned that women for whom estrogen is the right treatment—and that's a lot of women—will shy away from it," she says. "I've said this a lot. They're not going to get the vaginal protection or the bone protection that they would get from hormones. But as soon as there's an effective nonhormonal treatment for hot flashes, women are going to demand it." She laughs. "And physicians are going to need to learn a little more about hot flashes."

That's not to say there isn't a role for fezolinetant, Maki adds. "There certainly is, particularly for women unable or unwilling to take hormones and perhaps also for older women—but we need to tailor our treatments to make sure that women are getting the best treatment option for their needs."

Yet another exciting nonhormonal medication in the pipeline, says Minkin, is a drug that's also under development by Bayer called **elinzanetant**, which she describes as a "cousin" to fezolinetant. "The mechanism is very similar, and works in the hypothalamus," explains Minkin. Both medications, she says, will be the new frontier of nonhormonal but effective prescription medications for hot flashes.

The more options we have to stop the volcanic eruptions, the better.

• • • •

My best friend, Julie, and I are spending a perfect day together in New York City, starting with the Metropolitan Museum. We meet at ten on the dot, to "beat the crowds." Now that our kids are older, we have vowed to spend more time together, as we did when we were in our early twenties.

"I love that we've come full circle, and now we can run around together like we used to," I tell her.

"Remember when we would just walk all over the city, talking and talking?" she says. "We can finally do that again."

Julie and I first met when we were twenty-two. We had both been invited to a weekend party in upstate New York and found ourselves on a hayride that everyone but us seemed to be exuberantly enjoying. When I spotted Julie's morose expression, which mirrored my own, I immediately scooched next to her and introduced myself.

We were now going through menopause together.

We've been meeting at the Met, our happy place, for three decades. I tell her about one of my favorite Met events ever, which I did a few years ago, called the Museum Workout, a dance class in the museum that took place in the morning before opening hours. In that magical hour, a small group of us followed two instructors as they danced through the Met's venerable and beguilingly empty hallways, stopping to do jumping jacks in front of a nude marble statue of Perseus accompanied by music from Sly and the Family Stone.

On this day, we're taking in a sumptuous exhibit of portraits from the Medici. "I love that people think the balls on the Medicis' coat of arms might be coins," say Julie. "It's like all the family wants people to know about them is 'we're rich.'"

I ask her what would be on her family crest. "A cocktail shaker," she says. "No, an ankle brace. What about you?"

"Probably the JCPenney slogan 'It's all inside' in Latin," I tell her. My father and grandfather devoted their entire working lives to JCPenney.

"So yesterday I googled 'do hot flashes burn calories,'" Julie says. "And it autofilled, so everyone else is wondering that, too. Mine are so bad right now. I have hot flashes galore."

"I googled that, too!" I tell her. "I did some research and the answer is no, unfortunately. It doesn't seem fair. Hot flashes ignite my rosacea. How about you?" Along with an aversion to hayrides and an affinity for bad eighties pop, rosacea is one the many things Julie and I have in common.

"Yes, and I'm getting acne, too. My dad asked me what the bumps on my face were, just like when I was in high school." We stop in front of an imperious-looking gent with a hand on his hip who is, I tell Julie, a dead ringer for David Schwimmer from *Friends.*

She points at the name of the artist: Rosso Fiorentino. "And look, his name is Ross-o."

I tell Julie I've made an appointment with my doctor to talk about hormone therapy and she nods. "I did, too. I'm seeing a menopause practitioner after you told me about them. My shrink recommended her. I have an appointment in two months."

I tell her I used to be wary of MHT, but the more research I do and the more experts I consult, the more reassured I am.

"Me too," she says. "I would never have considered it, but then I read that taking it before sixty is fine. I said to my aunt Mattie that

I was thinking of taking it because my hot flashes were so bad, and she said, 'Big deal! We all had them.' Thanks!"

We move on to a somber, red-clad Giovanni de' Medici. We're trying to be appreciative of the art, like grown-ups, but our newfound freedom is making us act like seventh graders.

"Jon Lovitz," we say at the same time, as people move away from us, annoyed.

• • • •

As for other nonhormonal medications for hot flashes, NAMS lists a number that are used off-label to treat flashes because they are shown to have some benefit. Along with the gabapentin mentioned earlier, they include the antidepressants citalopram, desvenlafaxine, and escitalopram; clonidine, a drug used to treat hypertension; clonazepam, a drug typically used for epilepsy and migraine; and oxybutynin, which is used to treat an overactive bladder.

For those who don't want to take any medication, a procedure known as a stellate ganglion block may be worth investigating. Used in pain medicine, it's an injection of a local anesthetic into the stellate ganglion sympathetic nerves in the neck. Stellate ganglion block was shown in a small trial to have some effect in reducing hot flashes (or what some, in an effort to put a positive spin on things, are calling "power surges").

"A stellate ganglion block is not a recognized therapy option, so it's considered experimental," says Shen. "It seems to last for a few months and then requires repeat treatments. But for a patient who has tried everything else, and cannot do hormone therapy, that has been helpful."

Many women have found relief from herbal products such as black cohosh, dong quai, evening primrose oil, wild yam, and red clover. Just know that according to the Mayo Clinic's website,

"My mom is eighty-three and she still has hot flushes. She just starts to sweat from the very top of her head. So there's parts of it that I feel don't ever go away. It's a way of life and you learn to live with it."

—Stevie Nicks

"scientific evidence on effectiveness is lacking, and some of these products may be harmful." (As supplements aren't classified as drugs, approval by the FDA isn't required, and manufacturers aren't held responsible for their safety or effectiveness.)

Anna Camille Moreno of Duke University Medical Center says that although numerous studies have concluded that supplements in general are no better than placebos, "I get why they're popular. They're easily available, and you can hear a podcast about a supplement and immediately go buy it."

But just because it's over the counter doesn't mean it's harmless and all natural, Moreno cautions. "I have seen the effects of some of those supplements," she says. And because they're not FDA-regulated, "some can literally be coming from some part of the world that you don't know anything about as far as ingredients."

Lauren Streicher of Northwestern University's Feinberg School of Medicine adds that most of these sorts of remedies have been shown not to work beyond the initial placebo effect. "When it comes to hot flashes, we know that there is a huge placebo effect, and the placebo effect is real," she says. "So for about twelve weeks, pretty much any product you believe in will reduce the severity and number of hot flashes and help you sleep. So it does make your hot flashes go away, but it's not sustainable."

Take black cohosh, Streicher continues, "which people talk about all the time. If you look at the studies on black cohosh that say that it works, none of the studies was more than twelve weeks long." To bypass the placebo effect, she explains, "you have to have a fifty-two-week study that says that black cohosh works. And *those* studies show that it doesn't work."

That hasn't stopped a lucrative industry from springing up, Streicher goes on, bolstered by testimonials and "secret proprietary ingredients that are often the equivalent of oregano." If the supplements have studies to back them up, she advises patients, look carefully at the research. "You read these ads for supplements and it will say, 'Five out of ten women say our blue lavender extract made their hot flashes go away,'" says Streicher.

"Well, if you look at the actual study, that often isn't a valid scientific study—it's a *marketing* study. They put ten women in a room, gave them the blue lavender extract, asked if their hot flashes were better, and seven said, 'Yeah, I think so.' That's not a study!"

Of course, if your herbal or natural remedy is quashing your hot flashes and you've cleared it with your doctor, I am delighted for you.

Some doctors do recommend certain herbal remedies. If you've found black cohosh helpful, Dr. Minkin suggests a brand called Remifemin, from Germany, where herbs are regulated, and which she frequently uses for her breast cancer patients who can't take hormones.

Many ob-gyns recommend a plant-derived supplement called Equelle. It's comprised of S-equol, a soy derivative that binds to some of the body's estrogen receptors so that it's able to mimic the effects of estrogen, thereby reducing the frequency and severity of hot flashes in several small studies. If you're going to take it, patience is required, because you must wait two to three months for optimum effect.

If Moreno's patients want to try herbal supplements, she has them look for brands that are certified by U.S. Pharmacopeia, or USP, a nonprofit third-party organization that sets what *Consumer Reports* experts say are the most widely accepted standards for supplements.

While I'm on the subject of herbs, a 2020 study of midlife women found that 27 percent were using cannabis to manage menopausal symptoms such as hot flashes and sleep. Cannabis has yet to be scientifically studied in any large-scale way for a number of reasons, including that cannabis laws vary from state to state and that the FDA considers cannabis a Schedule 1 drug, defined as having "no currently accepted medical use" and the "highest potential for abuse." Mustering up clinical trials on cannabis, therefore, is a challenge.

But I do hear enthusiastic anecdotal evidence from many, many women in menopause that it helps. "Nothing else has worked for my joint pain in my hips and back except my CBD gummies," proclaims a former coworker. "Best thing for anxiety, a hell of a lot better than Celexa ever was," says another friend.

Given that many women appear to be self-dosing, research is vital. In a 2021 review in *Journal of Obstetrics and Gynaecology Canada,* Dr. Javier Mejia-Gomez and his colleagues scrutinized the published data on the effects of cannabis use in peri- and postmenopausal women. They came up with only a small handful of studies; not one was conducted by a group of menopause specialists.

In the Mature Women's Health and Menopause Clinic at Mount Sinai Hospital in Toronto where Mejia-Gomez works, he and his colleagues often see patients who are using cannabis either alone or as a complement of MHT, mainly for management of insomnia, pelvic pain, and anxiety.

"Due to the lack of research and evidenced-based medicine on this subject, it's hard for us to accurately counsel our patients," he laments. "If, as a society, we want to use cannabis to treat menopause efficiently and safely, then we need clear and consistent guidelines for physicians, decision-makers, and patients."

Northwestern University's Lauren Streicher, who writes about her ongoing research on menopause symptoms and cannabis in her excellently titled book *Hot Flash Hell,* says that her message to fellow gynecologists is "I'm not saying that you should recommend cannabis, because we don't have the data. But please acknowledge that your patients are using it, and know something about it so that you can start the conversation about options that we *do* know something about. Because women are using cannabis in droves. In droves! They're smoking it, putting it on their avocado toast, and putting it on their vulva."

If you're going to use it to alleviate menopause symptoms, she says, "know that it's not risk-free, start low and go slow, and think about using a tincture, which is measurable." (Streicher devotes a whole chapter to cannabis in *Hot Flash Hell*, along with detailed dosage guidelines.)

• • • •

Aside from herbs, there are plenty of lifestyle changes that have been shown to douse the flames.

Know your triggers, for starters. The most common, according to the Cleveland Clinic, are caffeine, alcohol, spicy foods, stress, and heat. There is no need to give them up entirely; just know to dial it back before, say, you're going on a date. Caffeine is a trigger for me, but there's no way I'm cutting down on my coffee, so I avoid it only before any occasion where I don't want my shiny, pulsating face and chest to frighten people. Nor am I eating a bland diet in order to dodge my other trigger, spicy foods—I'll just avoid jalapeños before meetings.

Regular exercise, one of the three pillars of health along with sleep and nutrition, can also help. Research presented at the NAMS annual conference in 2021 suggests that too many hours on the couch can increase nighttime hot flashes. That doesn't mean you have to leap up and immediately go out for a run, said Dr. Sarah

Witkowski, an exercise physiologist at Smith College and coauthor of the study. "Interrupting sedentary behavior is as easy as just getting up and moving around a bit."

If you smoke, now is the time to try to quit. I am not being cavalier about this and know full well how horrendously difficult it is—my mother said giving up her decades-long Kools habit was tougher than childbirth. But when women do manage to quit, studies show their hot flashes are less intense and less frequent.

Paced breathing, or slow, controlled deep respiration sustained for a specific period, has been shown to help dial back the severity and frequency of hot flashes, according to NAMS. The original natural remedy, it's free, can be used anytime, and couldn't be easier.

Deep breathing delivers a boatload of benefits for menopausal women. Several studies show it brings down levels of cortisol, the stress hormone, and does it fast. A 2017 study published in the journal *Frontiers in Psychology* found that diaphragmatic breathing enhanced the subjects' brain cognition and "significantly increased sustained attention." It has also been shown to reduce chronic pain in midlife women, so it can help with those newly aching joints.

When Gabriella Espinosa, a renowned London yoga, breathwork, and menopausal wellness instructor, entered perimenopause, she found that having a regular breath practice "gave me a sense of control, knowing that relief was not far away," she says. "When I felt a hot flash coming on, I knew I had a resource to anchor me so that I wouldn't spin off into a stress response, making things worse."

Engaging in breath practices, says Espinosa, reduces the neurochemicals produced by a stress response in the moment a hot flash comes on, helping to lower blood pressure, tamp down anxiety, and promote relaxation. Menopause can also be a time, Espinosa says, when women feel disconnected from their bodies, and frustrated with the lack of control they have with symptoms they experience. "Just a few minutes of breathwork has the power to shift the way you respond to discomfort in the moment and helps reconnect you with a sense of self and presence."

With paced breathing, she says, "you fully engage the stomach, abdominal muscles, and diaphragm. Your lower belly should expand with each outward breath. When you breathe normally, you are taking about twelve to fourteen breaths per minute. In paced breathing, you're taking only six or seven breaths a minute."

To start, sit upright. Place one hand on your abdomen and take a few diaphragmatic breaths, allowing your belly to bellow on the inhale and float back toward your spine on the exhale. Become aware of the physical sensations in your body, notice your thoughts without judgment, and softly repeat to yourself the comforting mantra "This too shall pass."

Begin to inhale deeply and softly through your nose on a count of four. Exhale slowly and gradually, releasing the breath through the nostrils on a count of eight ("or less, if this feels too long," she says). Repeat six to seven breaths for the next minute and stay with the practice for five to ten minutes, or as long as the hot flash lasts.

Espinosa's method has been tremendously helpful for me. I used to go rigid and quietly freak out when I felt a flash on the horizon. Now I lean into it, let it envelop me, and focus on breathing through it, which I've found does indeed make it recede faster. While I'm breathing, I've also been trying some positive self-talk, phrases like *You'll get through this.* An easy way to practice self-talk is simply to treat yourself the way you would a good friend or loved one. Be gentle and encouraging, rather than catastrophizing (*oh my god, what the hell is happening?*) or unkind (*whoa, you look like Mount Vesuvius about to blow*).

Positive self-talk is also a quick way to ramp down anxiety; a

2020 Iranian study found that positive self-talk was a useful coping strategy in stressful situations. When I'm talking to myself, I also use the word *you* when addressing myself (as in *you got this*). I picked up this technique from a 2017 study in the *Journal of Personality and Social Psychology*. Researchers found that when participants used *you* or their own names in positive self-talk rather than *I*, they were less anxious and stressed.

Finally, if you're experiencing night sweats, stash a spray bottle by your bed, such as the godsend Hot Flash Cooling Mist from a company called Pause Well-Aging (why didn't someone invent this sooner?), which I now keep on my nightstand.

Some women start wearing lighter pajamas to bed, but I soon got tired of wrenching them off in the middle of the night. Now, to make things simple and get immediate relief, I sleep commando. To hell with it.

· Chapter 5 ·

I Didn't Get Any Sleep, But I Did Catch Up on My Brooding

Why You Must Protect Your Rest

A few weeks after I meet Julie at the Met, we have another rendezvous, this time at Bloomingdale's in midtown Manhattan, where we are maintaining yet another thirty-year tradition of meeting for lunch at department stores, which we find both festive and comfortingly retro.

As we browse the perfume counters before heading upstairs to the restaurant, Forty Carrots, I realize that one of the few things I don't know about Julie is what perfume she wore as a teen in the eighties.

"I wore two Ralph Lauren perfumes," said Julie, picking up a bottle and giving it a delicate sniff. "One was called Tuxedo, and one was called . . ." She paused. "I don't know. Saddle?"

I nod. "That sounds like peak Ralph. Wait, was there such a thing as Saddle perfume?"

She thinks for a minute. "No. It was Lauren. I wore all Ralph's makeup, too. That was the lipstick Molly Ringwald put on in *The Breakfast Club* when Judd Nelson slow-clapped." She consulted her phone. "'Ralph Lauren Tuxedo was launched in 1979 as the evening fragrance of a true femme fatale,'" she reads aloud, then shakes her head. "When you're sixteen, you need an 'evening fragrance,' right?"

I tell her I wore Love's Baby Soft in my early teen years, then switched in my late teens to my own "evening" fragrance, Scoundrel perfume, after being intrigued by a TV commercial starring Joan Collins. "I took up Charlie perfume, too, which I felt was sophisticated."

We both break into the Charlie theme song. "Kinda young, kinda now—Charlie! Kinda free, kinda wow!" We both watched tons of TV as kids. At the restaurant, we are handed a menu that reads: *After a shopping spree at Bloomingdale's 59th Street, is there a more perfect way to unwind than grabbing a bite at Forty Carrots?*

No, there is not, we both agree. "I like that department-store restaurants still exist," says Julie. "It makes me feel like the world is okay. Now, let me see." She studies the menu. "How about starters from the Carrot Patch? There's no kale anywhere on this menu, thank god. Oh, look at the Flagship Trio platter—that's got a scoop of tuna salad, chicken salad, and egg salad. With a scoop of frozen yogurt! So, four scoops."

I decide on a tuna sandwich, while Julie opts for the Forty Carrots Chopped Salad.

"I think we need to have the frozen yogurt for dessert," says Julie. She points to the menu, which reads: *Find out what all the fuss is about!* "I want to see for myself what the fuss is about."

Bloomingdale's is our safe place, where nothing bad can happen.

Julie has memories of going to Forty Carrots with her mom in White Plains, New York. I feel sentimental about department stores because my dad managed various JCPenneys, so I spent a lot of time as a kid following Dad around as he chatted with shoppers and employees, always on the alert for problems he could step in and solve.

For both of us, that feeling of safety is rooted in childhood memories of having a grown-up in charge, of still being naive as to how unsafe any place could be.

As we dig into our lunch, I tell Julie that when Dad retired, I was living in Koreatown in New York and working as an editor at *Rolling Stone.* Sometimes when I would grow weary of trying to be hip, I'd take a train to the Short Hills Mall in my home state of New Jersey and proceed directly to Bloomingdale's linens section on the basement floor.

There, I would drift around for a long time, touching various towels and wishing I could crawl into the display beds piled with pillows and take a long nap. The orderly folded sheets in rainbow colors comforted me, as did the atmosphere of quiet and calm. The staff in Linens was always a little older—I sensed management thought, *They've done their time. Let's give them a break and put them in Linens, where there's not much action and no loud dance music like in Women's Contemporary Apparel.*

"I didn't sleep well last night," Julie says. "Again. I have a hot flash every hour, which wakes me up. Also, sometimes cold flashes. Are they a thing?"

They are, I tell her.

"I take a lot of things to make sure I sleep, like my pot gummies and Klonopin," says Julie. "But all of that can only help you fall asleep—you have to *stay* asleep, which seems to be a whole other thing when you're in menopause."

She sighs. "I was just in the elevator of my building this morning and the sweat was dripping down my forehead. I need to sleep.

"Did I have night sweats?
I was literally sleeping with
[a bag of] frozen peas in between
my breasts and frozen peas
behind my neck."

—Rosie O'Donnell

I feel hungover when I don't. I can't wait to see if I can do hormone therapy."

"My mom just told me she was on Premarin for ten years," I said. "I had no idea."

"Has your mother shrunk at all, by the way?" said Julie. "My mother was, like, five-ten, and now she's shorter than me." We signal the waiter to order frozen yogurt.

• • • •

Insomnia, studies show, is considerably more common in women. Throughout all stages of life, women report getting insufficient sleep more often than men, finds a 2018 study in *Clinical Pulmonary Medicine*. The demographic skew is thanks to physiological and hormonal changes during adolescence, the menstrual cycle, pregnancy, perimenopause, and menopause—not to mention issues such as "childcare responsibilities, work-life balance, the caregiver role for the elderly, and stress." Sound familiar?

Some sleep problems, the authors note, such as insomnia, hypersomnia (insomnia is the inability to fall asleep, hypersomnia is the inability to stay awake), and restless legs syndrome, are also more common in women.

I've been keeping a sleep diary, and I'm up an average of five times a night, I tell Dr. Wen Shen at Johns Hopkins. "It makes so many of my patients wrung out and irritable, and apt to go into a rage," says Shen. "I've had patients come to me who say they haven't slept in years. Years! They tell me that they don't even recognize themselves anymore."

UC Berkeley sleep scientist Matthew Walker, author of *Why We Sleep*, often says that no aspect of our biology is unscathed by sleep deprivation. We all know by now that chronic sleep loss wreaks havoc on your health—not only making you confused and irritable, but driving up the risks of developing heart disease, stroke, high blood pressure, and type 2 diabetes, according to the CDC. It messes with memory, mood, and metabolism.

Growing research even suggests that sleep loss during menopause—what author Samantha Irby has called "menopause o'clock"—is the culprit behind menopausal weight gain, which usually collects around your middle.

Thanks to hot flashes and night sweats, among other reasons, many women in menopause tend to wake up repeatedly in the night, says Harvard's Dr. Hadine Joffe. She and her team describe these periods of wakefulness as WASO, short for wakefulness after sleep onset. When your sleep cycles are constantly breaking up, you can miss the deep type of sleep in non-REM, or rapid eye movement, that is so restorative (with non-REM, there is both light and deep sleep). In a typical night's sleep, the brain goes back and forth between REM and non-REM sleep. During REM sleep, your brain wave activity ramps up as it processes information, experiences, and emotions that it picked up that day, committing some to memory and discarding others. Major muscles that you normally control during sleep, such as the ones in your arms and legs, can't move in the REM phase, becoming so zonked that they are temporarily paralyzed.

Missing this crucial restorative non-REM deep sleep phase can leave you feeling as tired during the day as having had short sleep. Surprisingly, it may be just as important for your health, says Joffe, to get even five hours of solid uninterrupted high-quality sleep versus eight or nine hours of splintered sleep.

"It's not just the total hours," Joffe says. "Meaning that you can't just say, 'Well, I was up several times last night, so I'm just going to sleep in until ten,'" says Joffe. "It's about having those consolidated deep patterns of sleep, and if you're constantly interrupting it, you never have that deep, *deep* sleep, and the restfulness that comes out of it." As rest is, again, one of the often-cited three pillars of health, Joffe says it's vital to ensure your sleep is consolidated.

At this point, most of us are aware of the edicts of good sleep hygiene: Keep screens out of the bedroom, as tempting as they may be; get up after twenty minutes of tossing and turning so you don't associate your bed with restlessness; try to get some exercise during the day; keep the bedroom dark and cool (60 to 65 degrees is the ideal temperature, per the Sleep Foundation).

Women in the menopause transition, says Joffe, should systematically go through their sleep habits and prune anything that interrupts their rest that they are able to control. You're already fighting a battle just to sleep during menopause, much less all the other factors that are siphoning off your slumber. Are you doomscrolling on your phone right before you turn out the light? Is your cat sleeping on your chest?

And it's not just consolidation of sleep that's vital, says Yu Fang, a researcher at the University of Michigan's Neuroscience Institute's Sen Lab. Keeping a regular sleep-wake schedule, she says, is an unappreciated factor that is as important for mental health as having enough sleep time. In a 2021 study whose subjects were first-year medical residents—a sleep-deprived group if ever there was one—Fang and her colleagues found that an irregular sleep schedule can increase a person's risk of depression as much as getting fewer hours of sleep overall.

Experts say that having a consistent waking time in particular, even on weekends, is one of the best ways to regulate our body's circadian rhythms, the 24-hour internal clock that is cued by light and dark. "That means getting up at the same time every day, no matter what time you fell asleep, no matter how crappy your sleep was," says Dr. Thurston.

I took Dr. Thurston's advice, and it was a game-changer for me. I decided to start going to bed at 10:40 P.M.—a little nutty, I know, but I found that's exactly when I started nodding off each night. I wake up each morning at 6:40 when my kid gets up for school—and now I do it on weekends, too. Is it rock 'n' roll? No. But this new habit has done more to regulate my sleep than anything else.

Another persistent thief of sleep is partners who snore. When my husband, Tom, had a particularly nasty bout of flu, I, a rabid germaphobe, asked him to sleep in the spare room. It was a revelation. While I was still waking up multiple times a night from hot flashes, I quickly realized that Tom's snoring, a succession of hog noises beginning with a series of staccato snorts, moving on to a midrange set of syncopated wheezes, and culminating in a high, prolonged porcine squeal, was consistently waking me up.

How disruptive can snoring get? When researchers measured the decibel levels of snorers in a 2020 study published in the journal *Sleep*, they found that 14 percent went over the 53-decibel level that's classified as *noise pollution*.

Even when people assume they get a better sleep when their partner is nearby, researchers from Ryerson University in Toronto have discovered otherwise. As Colleen Carney, director of Ryerson's Sleep and Depression Laboratory, told the CBC, "People will say they sleep better [together], but when we actually monitor their brains, we see that their brain is not getting into deeper stages of sleep because they're continuously being woken up by movement or sound." (Not their *own* movement or sound.)

One solution that's gaining more traction is getting what's called a "sleep divorce," in which couples maintain the relationship but sleep apart, either part time or full time. It's not as uncommon as you might think: a 2017 National Sleep Foundation survey found that nearly one in four couples retire to separate bedrooms. Home builders the Toll Brothers cite an increasing demand for what is known as dual primary bedrooms.

Some menopausal women tell me they sleep with their partner on alternate nights; others share a bedroom only on weekends. Some have pre-bedtime rituals where they wind down together in one bed; then one partner will discreetly slip away. Yes, they may miss a little snuggling, but in the words of renowned sex therapist Esther Perel, "What's the last thing you stroke at night before you fall asleep? What's the first thing you touch in the morning when you wake up? Be honest. Is it your phone?"

I'm not ready for a full sleep divorce, but if there is any chance that Tom could interrupt my sleep, I ask him to bunk down in the spare room. That includes his late-night "tournaments" with his Fortnite Over 40 group—yes, this is real, formed by midlife gamers fed up with of being scorned and trash-talked by younger and more adept players—or his IRL weekly soccer game (usually followed by beers). When he stumbles in after a night of gaming or carousing, he inevitably wakes me up.

I tell Dr. Thurston that I feel a twinge of guilt when I ask Tom to sleep in a separate room. "Do it," she says. "*Do it.* Sleep is important to mental health, to cognition, to the brain. We have a paper showing that women who are waking up a lot during the night have more vascular damage in the brain. This is all really, really important."

• • • •

I know that for many going through a rough menopause, a cocktail can be the elixir of life, but alcohol can be a stealthy robber of good-quality sleep. A towering pile of studies confirms that booze interferes with deep sleep, yet it remains one of the most popular sleep aids in the United States—used by an estimated one-fifth of Americans with chronic insomnia.

Alcohol, which depresses the central nervous system, does have sedative qualities that may bring on sleep faster. But people who drink before bed often experience more awakenings and less of that delicious restorative non-REM sleep, as their liver begins metabolizing the alcohol in the second half of the night. If your rest is fragmented by hot flashes and night sweats, alcohol may splinter it further.

I've interviewed many sleep experts over the years. (For health journalists, sleep loss is a so-called evergreen story, reliably popular with readers no matter what the news hook is.) Many have told me that their patients who believe they have an insomnia disorder are in fact tipping back booze too close to bedtime.

To discern if alcohol is actually the culprit, they tell their patients to see if they can refrain for two weeks, while keeping a sleep diary. The results can be an eye-opener.

If you can't bear the thought of giving up alcohol and believe life is to be lived, experts say to try to put down the Pinot four hours before heading off to bed. "I mean, I like my wine," says Dr. Thurston, "but we know that we become more sensitive to alcohol as we age, and it really starts to screw up your sleep."

I'm more inclined to pop melatonin supplements, and I'm not alone, as the number of Americans using melatonin has quadrupled in the past two decades. In some countries, such as England, melatonin is only available by prescription, but it's readily available over the counter in the United States, where even kids can take L'il Critters' 1.5 milligram melatonin gummies (in a peach flavor that is "soooo yummy!").

Melatonin, sometimes called the Dracula hormone because it

emerges at night, is produced naturally by your brain to cue your body for sleep and gradually power down. During the menopause transition, your body's production of melatonin, like estrogen, drops.

For some, it doesn't work, or makes them feel too sludgy the next morning, but for others, melatonin is sent from heaven on a pink cloud. Many people take 5 milligrams or even 10, but experts caution to start low, at .5 milligram. While you may be tempted to jack up the dosage, more is not necessarily better: MIT researchers found that a mere .3 milligram of melatonin nightly before bed helped adults over fifty who were plagued by insomnia to sleep through the night.

An even better combination is melatonin with a consistent bedtime, according to a 2018 Australian study. When researchers had subjects take .5 milligram of melatonin an hour before turning in, along with going to bed at a set time, the participants dropped off to sleep 34 minutes earlier and had greater sleep time and fewer sleep disturbances.

Others love their CBD gummies to bring on slumber. About a third of 1,500 women surveyed in a 2021 Canadian study reported using cannabis, most often in the form of edibles, for menopause symptoms such as lack of sleep. There's not yet a lot of research yet on menopausal insomnia and CBD—but again, given how many women are self-diagnosing and tossing it back, there should be.

My friend Nia takes 50 milligrams of CBD every night. "Two gummies to sleep and chill," she says. "It's like everything you like about weed, without getting high. I know vaping is quicker, but I'm okay with timing it to take effect, because I feel like gummies are safer." (This, according to *Consumer Reports*, is true: when some solvents in vaping oils are heated to high temperatures, they can convert to carcinogens such as formaldehyde.)

Many people swear by magnesium's soporific effects, although a

"I will wake up just soaking, like the whole sheets, the pillowcase. And then I'm too lazy to do anything about it. I have friends that get up and change, but I just sleep in it. And then I wake up freezing cold. It's just a good time."

—author Glennon Doyle

recent meta-analysis found there isn't solid research behind it. Scientists aren't sure why it might work; one theory is that magnesium deficiencies disrupt levels of sleep-inducing hormones. There are several forms of magnesium; if you plan on taking it, the Cleveland Clinic recommends 200 milligrams of magnesium glycinate or 200 milligrams of magnesium citrate. Avoid magnesium oxide, instructs the clinic's website with what I interpret as sly humor, "which is a stool softener and probably much less helpful for your insomnia."

If hot flashes and night sweats are your primary sleep stealer, consider hormone therapy. A 2017 review in the journal *Sleep Science* called it "the most recommendable and well-established" treatment for hot flashes and their related sleep disturbances. "In women with hot flashes who go on estrogen, it does improve their sleep," confirms Joffe, "although we don't really know if it's because we're treating the hot flashes and they are therefore sleeping better, or if it's something more direct." Research shows that progesterone, as part of MHT, shortens the time it takes to fall asleep, lessens awakenings during the night, and increases total sleep time.

Taking a pill may not always be necessary. Work with your circadian rhythms by remembering a simple rule: more light energy during the day, less at night. Go outside and view some natural light, even for just two minutes, within an hour of waking, and do it once again in the late afternoon prior to sunset to cue your brain that it's time to start winding down—again, even for just two minutes, but preferably ten.

Dim the lights from ten P.M. on, and avoid turning on any overhead lights, which Stanford University neuroscientist Dr. Andrew Huberman says activates melanopsin cells in your eyes that tell your brain and body when light is present (*sun's out, let's go!*). The lower your lights are physically in the room, Dr. Huberman has said, the better.

One of the best ways to bring on sleep, say many experts, is cognitive behavioral therapy for insomnia, or CBT-I. It's a structured program that helps you stop nighttime ruminating and enables you to identify and replace sleep-sabotaging behaviors with slumber-promoting habits. The beauty of CBT-I is that unlike the temporary fix of a pill, it helps people overcome the underlying *causes* of sleep troubles "and really helps you find ways to release the ruminative thoughts," says Dr. Rebecca Thurston. "We can't suppress them, so it's more of a releasing, and giving yourself reassuring statements like *It's going to be okay, I've gone through this before, I can address these thoughts tomorrow,* and deep breathing. You work with people to develop those cognitive strategies that help them let the rumination go."

The American Academy of Sleep Medicine has a searchable database of accredited sleep centers and practitioners that offer CBT-I (sleepeducation.org). And as with a certified menopause practitioner, you don't have to go forever. "It's safer than medication, it's less addictive, and it's durable," says Thurston. "You see CBT-I really improving sleep for the long term."

The research behind it is solid, too, adds Dr. Joffe. "We did a clinical trial for CBT-I, with women who had hot flashes and sleep disturbances, and it was hugely effective for their insomnia symptoms," she says. Further, "when we did meta-analyses and looked at all of our trials, we found it really is the frontline treatment for chronic insomnia."

Joffe says that science-backed sleep-enhancing apps can also be effective. Many doctors recommend ShutEye, Sleepio, and my favorite, CBT-i Coach, a free app developed by Stanford School of Medicine in collaboration with the federal government. It has breathing tools and a sleep diary, and it gives you alternate thoughts when brooding starts to creep in, such as: *Even if I miss some sleep, I will be able to function. I can tolerate this. I will survive even if I don't sleep at all tonight. I don't have to feel comfortable all the time. This is another challenge that I will figure out and face.*

These can replace my ruminative thoughts, such as *Is Sarah out to get me? What happens if my mother's vertigo gets worse? Should I have included a smiley-face emoji on that text I sent to the boss? What if I didn't lock up downstairs and left the door open and the cat gets out? What if the cat gets out and runs in front of a car? What if I drive the car in the morning, and my own lost cat rushes out in front of my car?*

Instead, I've learned to sub in helpful mantras such as: *I have done my best today. I am safe and calm here in my bed. I am at peace. I am going to sleep now so that I can heal my mind and body.*

Mindful deep breathing, as it does with hot flashes, has also been shown to set off a cascade of physiological responses that hastens sleep. One popular formula among sleep specialists is the following: Lie down and put one hand on your chest, and one on your belly. Inhale through your nose for 4 counts. Hold for 7 counts, and exhale though your mouth for 8 counts.

Stressful thoughts spike our heart rate and cortisol levels, a fight-or-flight response deeply rooted in primordial human responses to danger, like harmful predators. "In today's world," as one sleep paper somewhat depressingly puts it, "the bear is always there."

Rafael Pelayo, a clinical professor in Stanford University's division of sleep medicine, has said that for many of us, the only time that we're alone with our thoughts is when we are in bed. If you find that your racing mind is keeping you awake, he recommends that you schedule some designated time in the evening away from your bed where you can be alone with your thoughts. I started taking an after-dinner walk to at least try to process some of the problems that arose during the day.

While most sleep research focuses on bedtime rumination about past events, bedtime worry about future events—the old "what did I forgot to do today that's going to screw up tomorrow?"—may also be important. Incomplete tasks cause a "high level of cognitive activation," according to one sleep paper.

Joffe tells patients to get a little notebook, preferably with a cover so you can't see what you write, and put it by your bed. "I call it the worry list book or the to-do list book," she says. "Write down your list during the day, or before bed. If you wake up in the middle of the night, you can then reassure yourself by thinking, 'I don't need to rehearse that, recite that, or ruminate on that. It's there, and I will get to it tomorrow.'" A 2018 study found that people who spent five minutes creating a to-do list before bed fell asleep faster than a control group.

Finally, once you've written down all your to-dos, the CBT-i app advises users to keep middle-of-the-night thoughts as soothingly mundane as possible.

I tell Julie this at Bloomingdale's and she laughs. "I don't have to try," she says. "I've pretty much got you covered when it comes to mundane thoughts."

"I guarantee mine are more boring," I say as I shovel in my frozen yogurt, which, as it turns out, is indeed "worth the fuss."

"Okay, let's have a contest," I say. Julie and I love contests, which usually involve trying to stump each other with random lyrics to eighties pop songs. (I once won with this one: "I've been funny, I've been cool with the lines." Hint: former *General Hospital* star.)

Julie goes first with her official entry for Who Had the Most Boring Thoughts Last Night.

"So, as you know, it took me forever to get new place mats," she begins.

I nod. We have had several extremely involved discussions about the place mats.

"I finally got some from Etsy from a Lithuanian woman, and they're very pretty, but when they showed up, they came with this letter written in calligraphy telling you how to handwash them."

"Calligraphy," I say, nodding gravely. "A red flag."

"Right? And it's this long process, like 'Fill a bowl with cold water, dunk them in gently,' and so on," says Julie, finishing up her frozen yogurt. "Last night at around three, I thought, *Do I pull the trigger and get more place mats?* That's what I was wrestling with. I don't want to spend more money, but I just want to throw my place mats in the washing machine."

She holds up her hand. "No, I have an even more boring one. I told you we have a new super in our building? His name is Elvis."

She signals for the check. "So I have a small light in my kitchen above the counter and it doesn't work. My old super, Ivan, could always get it to work, but I feel like I can't call Elvis yet because he's new. You know? Like, while he's settling in, it should only be an emergency."

I decide I'll submit two entries, too. "I was up last night thinking about how my mother has vertigo and how my neighbor said that an ear, nose, and throat doctor can take this special vibrating tool, put it next to your head, and turn it on. She said the vibrations will shake loose these crystals in your inner ear that supposedly cause vertigo. I was wondering if I could take this really powerful back massager that I have and just sort of stick it on my mom's head and turn it on."

Julie considers this. "It might. It just might."

I submit entry number two. "You know those fried onions that you put on green bean casseroles at Thanksgiving? I have some leftover ones, and I was musing about what else I could put them on. Soup, maybe?"

Julie shrugs. "Or you could just eat them out of the bag."

"True."

After a long debate, we decide that the Most Mundane Thought contest is a draw.

· Chapter 6 ·

50, Shades of Gray

Why Am I Losing the Hair on My Head and Gaining It on My Chin?

At the close of 2021, a *New York Times* article appeared entitled "Why Do Women Sprout Chin Hairs as They Age?" It was quickly flooded with nearly a thousand comments, many of which had me nodding.

There was one comment that resonated most: *I have found my tribe.*

During the menopause transition, says Beverly Hills ob-gyn Thaïs Aliabadi, a woman's body stops circulating estrogen but continues to circulate the same amounts of androgens like testosterone. "The imbalance of hormones causes the appearance of some male secondary sex characteristics, like coarse facial hair," she says.

As the balance of hormones in your body shifts, the hair on your head can become sparser, while the hair on your face can grow more prevalent. This sudden migration can take the form of peach fuzz that covers your complexion like a low-pile carpet or thick dark hairs that spring up on areas of your face where the hair follicles are especially androgen sensitive, like the upper lip and chin.

While, as Aliabadi points out, "there's nothing wrong or unhealthy about a few extra chin hairs," they can be unsettling, especially when they seemingly sprout half an inch overnight. Inevitably, you will become aware of their wiry presence when you are out somewhere in a public place, perhaps enjoying lunch with friends, when your fingertips absently brush your chin. You feel a novel outgrowth and suddenly wish your fingers were a pair of tweezers. You can see your friend's lips moving, but all you can think is *chin hair chin hair long thick chin hair.*

I've often thought that some enterprising jewelry maker should craft a pendant with a pair of tiny tweezers concealed inside for surreptitious plucking. (And I now keep a pair in the storage compartment of my car, because, like one *New York Times* commenter pointed out, I've found that the car's visor mirror is ruthless.)

Options abound to remove the bristly buggers. Along with plucking, waxing, threading, and sugaring can reduce hair growth by weakening the follicle. Like improper lawn weeding, treatments like dermaplaning and depilatory creams remove every last hair but don't do anything at the root.

A prescription cream called Vaniqa makes hair grow in more slowly. (No generic is available, and it's not cheap, so Vaniqa might be best for small areas like the new soul patch you've sprouted.) For permanent hair removal, lasers and electrolysis banish hair by damaging the follicle so it never grows back.

And my friends and I now have a mantra that we call I Have Your Chin: if you see something, say something.

• • • •

During the menopause transition, your appearance, in one way or another, is going to change—your skin, your hair, your body. I'll tell you why it's happening and what you can do about it—*if* you want to. The goal here is to do whatever makes you feel reasonably like yourself during this natural life process. If weaving your chin hairs into a braid and affixing a bead to the end or declaring "If it's gray, it stays" enables you to come back to yourself, that is absolutely what you should do.

It may not seem like it sometimes, but our culture's perception of what a fifty-year-old woman looks like has changed fairly radically in the past few decades. After the 2020 Super Bowl, a meme quickly circulated around Jennifer Lopez's electrifying halftime performance. It was a split screen showing Blanche Devereaux of *The Golden Girls* with a fusty hairdo and old-fashioned sweater ("50 in 1985") and a lithe Lopez, swinging around a pole in a tiny sequined jumpsuit ("50 in 2020").

I get the point that the meme's creators were making, but there is not a thing wrong with looking like Blanche, nor should there be any pressure on any woman in midlife to look like Lopez. (I once interviewed her and can attest that in person, her otherworldly beauty is so distracting that at one point I slurringly called her "Jeffer.")

I once had hair as thick and glossy as Jeffer's. No longer. One day as I'm exiting the shower, I look down and note with dismay that a large hamster-like ball of my hair has collected in the drain. I brush my hair, zero in on my suddenly wide part with alarm, and immediately phone my sister Dinah. I don't even say hello, which I feel you can do with family members. Dinah is more affable than I am, and likes to open with normal, polite questions, such as 'How was your weekend?" but she has adapted to my quirks. "You're almost in menopause, right?" I asked. "Is your hair falling out, by chance? My part is getting bigger. Is yours?"

"Yes, yes, and yes," she says. "I noticed it about six months ago. It got thinner, especially near the hairline at the top of my forehead."

"Mine's more at the crown," I tell her. "I just noticed I'm getting patchy. No one wants a patchy head."

"They do not," Dinah affirms.

I conference in my sister Heather, ask her the same question. "Oh, god, it's terrible," she says. "I feel like it's thinning at the top of my forehead, which is really freaky."

"I was just telling Jancee that," says Dinah.

"And it's drier and breaks more easily," says Heather. "I usually end up sort of foofing my hair a little forward."

"'Foofing' means arranging, I take it?" Dinah asks.

"Yes," says Heather. "So it covers the thin patches."

My sisters and I are not alone in our hair travails. In a study published in the journal *Menopause* in 2022, Thai researchers examined the scalps of over 200 menopausal women and found that more than half of them experienced thinning hair, a common condition called female pattern hair loss, or FPHL.

While it's unclear exactly why menopausal women's hair starts to thin, the research suggested that plummeting estrogen levels may affect hair follicles, where estrogen receptors are present. Complex biologic, genetic, and hormone effects cause the follicles to shrink, causing hair to be finer, and the hair's growing phase gets shorter, says Alison Bruce, a dermatologist at the Mayo Clinic in Jacksonville, Florida. There's also a genetic component, she says.

While receding hair among men is more normalized, it can be a shock when women notice a dwindling ponytail or more hair collecting in their brushes. I tell Bruce about my capacious new hair part. Typically, with FPHL, she explains, "the frontal hairline stays the same, but the part is wider, and there's thinning in the center at the top of the scalp, kind of like a Christmas tree," she says. Maybe I can wear a star on top of my head.

Patients also tell Bruce that they'll notice that "their scalp is getting sunburned and that didn't happen before. It's really distressing for women."

Fortunately, hair loss can be treated. First, says New York City dermatologist Macrene Alexiades, see your physician to ensure that there isn't an underlying cause. While hair loss may be commonplace during the menopausal transition, it could also be caused by conditions such as an autoimmune disease, thyroid issues, or anemia. "I do a full blood workup for my patients," says Alexiades. "See a doctor, don't self-medicate."

If you get a clean bill of health, the simplest solution to kick-start growth is 5 percent minoxidil, known by its brand name Rogaine, which Bruce says is effective in about two out of three people that use it. (Stick with it, she adds, as noticeable results may take at least three months.)

Spironolactone, a daily oral blood pressure medication that's used off-label for hormonal hair loss, can restore hair growth and prevent hair loss from getting worse, according to the American Academy of Dermatology (AAD), by blocking the effects of testosterone in the body. A 2020 study from the *Journal of the American Academy of Dermatology* found that women who used it for six months saw significant improvement. As is true with all drugs, there are side effects: spironolactone is a diuretic, so it can cause dehydration-induced dizziness, for starters.

A promising nondrug option is platelet-rich plasma (PRP) injections, in which the patient's blood is drawn, spun in a centrifuge, and injected in the scalp to stimulate hair growth. "As we age, we're

"You know what? Menopause is hell, Jimmy. Menopause is a dark hole. Okay? That's what menopause is. And that's where I'm at right now."

—Viola Davis, responding to Jimmy Kimmel's question "What is menopause?" on *Jimmy Kimmel Live* not getting the blood circulation to our scalp that we did, and PRP really works," says Alexiades. In Bruce's Regenerative Medicine clinic, patients have to endure forty to fifty injections, but she says they may see up to a 15 percent improvement; pair PRP with minoxidil, as Bruce's research has shown, and results can be even better.

There is some data that suggests scalp massage can help. A 2019 study published in the journal *Dermatology and Therapy* showed that a twenty-minute scalp massage, administered twice daily, aided hair growth. After six months, a full 69 percent of participants reported losing less hair, which was documented by photos. Scalp massage is free, effective, and it feels good—a magical combination. (If you don't want to use your fingers for a massage, manual massagers, often made of silicone, are available on Amazon for a few bucks.)

Bruce and other dermatologists say there isn't yet good data on ingestible collagen's effect on hair and nails, although anecdotal evidence may be encouraging. As for other supplements, iron is important for hair growth, and iron supplementation, according to the Cleveland Clinic, can help stop hair loss. One of the first things hair clinics often do is screen for deficiencies, as many women have low levels of iron—especially those who are vegetarians. A 2018 review of thirteen studies in the *American Journal of Lifestyle Medicine* found that vegetarian women in particular had a "high prevalence of depleted iron stores."

Treat hair gently and try deep conditioners if it's newly dry and frizzy, keeping in mind that loss of estrogen and progesterone decreases the production of sebum, the natural oil your scalp makes that coats hair and gives it shine. Hair volumizing powders add life to a sparse scalp by pumping up the volume. Comprised of a dry formula that contains bulking ingredients like rice powder or silica silylate, it's sprayed or sprinkled on your roots to add instant texture and bulk. A hairstylist can do a volume-enhancing cut; a colorist can deploy a technique called color contouring, in which strategically placed highlights add the perception of dimension to flat-looking locks by using shadows and light.

• • • •

Let's move on to weight.

Dr. Mary Jane Minkin says that while some experts dispute that menopause is associated with weight gain, most people do in fact put on weight during this time of life. The average gain during the menopause transition, she says, is five to eight pounds.

During the menopause transition, adds Dr. Makeba Williams, weight in general can be tougher to lose. Williams, who is in her mid-forties, calls herself a "Peloton OG" who started riding when she was thirty-eight. "I've watched my own body change over the last couple of years," she says. "Lately I've been wondering if Peloton changed the metric, or, you know, if my bike is old." She laughs. "Nope! I'm just not as efficient. Now I get what my patients are saying and can show greater empathy when they tell me, 'I'm doing as much exercise as I can, and I don't see the scale moving.'"

One significant contributing factor to menopausal weight gain that many people don't consider, says Dr. Lauren Streicher of Northwestern University, is hot flashes. "The elevation in cortisol that occurs during hot flashes slows down your metabolism, making it harder to lose weight," she says. "A small transient rise in cortisol doesn't cause problems, but if it's chronically, consistently elevated, there's an increase in blood sugar levels and appetite.

"When a woman comes into our center and announces that she gained twenty pounds since menopause and can't take it off," says Streicher, "our first question is 'Are you having hot flashes?' And our second question is 'Are you sleeping?' Because lack of sleep is associated with weight gain."

Streicher maintains that it's not the lack of estrogen that leads to weight gain in menopause. "It's the hot flashes, it's the elevation in cortisol, it's your sleep getting screwed up so you make different food choices, and are too tired to exercise. I make the case that you've got to get rid of the hot flashes if you want to lose the weight."

Even if menopause doesn't add any pounds, you'll likely see a change in where your body fat is stored—which is normal. As the NAMS website relays, "Although menopause may not be directly associated with weight gain, it may be related to changes in body composition and fat distribution. Several studies have shown that perimenopause, independent of age, is associated with increased fat in the abdomen as well as decreased lean body mass. This suggests that menopause plays a role in many midlife women's transition from a pear-shape body (wide hips and thighs) to an apple-shaped body (wide waist and belly)."

While I read this and imagine my butt slowly drifting across my body like an iceberg, and lodging, finally, on my stomach, I do find this information incredibly freeing. Those extra pounds that have accumulated around your middle are *not* because you let yourself go or because you're "lazy." It's biology. It's a physiological change. You can do a thousand abdominal crunches a day and that gut may stay stubbornly put. (There's scant evidence that spot reduction works, anyway.) It happens to most of us, it might never go away, and *it's okay.*

I gained around ten pounds during menopause, and it went straight to my middle—to the point where none of my pants fit, except a few very loose, forgiving "joggers" that have yet to see a jog. A year after my weight gain, I still couldn't stuff myself into a single pair of those pants. To say that they ceased to spark joy was an understatement—I felt like they were hanging in silent judgment in my closet. I phone up Jamie Medley, a chic, exuberant fashion influencer from Richmond, Virginia, beloved by menopausal women on Instagram, and ask her what I should do.

"Donate them," she says immediately. "It's been a year. Start anew! Add some color! Accept what you've got, and work with what you have." Medley, now in her sixties, tells me that she, too, gained weight in her middle during menopause—and it never came off. "I used to be a size 4 or 6 and now I'm a 10 or a 12," she says. "I don't pay attention to a number. Who knows but you? Who is looking at it but you?"

Medley's number one tip for her followers is to buy clothes in a larger size and get them taken in. "The older you get, the more you need a good seamstress," she says. "Then your clothes look more expensive, and like they were tailor made for you."

Your weight may be staying where it is, but there are countless benefits to maintaining an exercise regimen. Lean muscle mass decreases with age as well as with estrogen loss, says Dr. Makeba Williams, "but muscle cells are much more efficient at burning calories than fat cells, so it's important to build lean muscle." Women over fifty also need lean muscle to stabilize their joints and maintain bone strength. Regular exercise helps stave off that decline.

If you've stopped moving—which happens so often in midlife when you're working or taking care of others—do your best to start again. "I stopped exercising when I had kids," says my friend Kathy. "Now that my youngest is in college, I try to be active. I do yardwork, because I have this insane impulse to be productive all the time, but I put on a podcast, so I'm not even thinking about it as I pick up sticks or whatever. And I find that the more exercise I do, the more energy I have. I think I have more energy now in my fifties than I did in my twenties, probably because I was hungover all the time—but still, that's been a nice surprise."

Try for muscle-strengthening activities to increase your lean body mass, such as weight training or push-ups, at least twice a week, says Camille Moreno at Duke University Medical Center.

Regular exercise is the closet equivalent to a magic pill. It helps ward off osteoporosis, diabetes, and heart disease. It lifts your mood by boosting levels of so-called happy chemicals like serotonin, and helps you sleep. The U.S. Department of Health recommends 2.5 hours to 5 hours a week of moderate to intense aerobic activity. And it doesn't need to be training for a triathlon, either: the USDH maintains that walking briskly qualifies. Bring a friend! Bring the dog!

Dog owners, by the way, have been shown to be much more likely to meet the standard exercise recommendation than those who don't have a canine—known by researchers as the "Lassie effect" for the lifesaving benefits of regular dog walking. "I'm not that motivated on my own," says my neighbor Tracey, "but I'll go out if my dog flops on the floor and looks at me accusingly."

As for an eating regimen, Chicago registered dietician Christy Brissette offers the sort of sensible advice that you would expect from an RD: Eat mindfully rather than thoughtlessly, and load up on vegetables. Go for slow-release complex carbs that don't cause your insulin levels to spike, she says, which leads to storing extra fat, especially around the belly, and get protein at every meal, which can help you keep the muscle you do have. And avoid dieting at all costs, Brissette says. "Research shows strict diets not only cause you to regain the weight once you go off them, but the weight you gain is going to be mostly abdominal fat."

A 2021 report in the journal *Critical Reviews in Food Science and Nutrition* recommends that physicians prescribe the Mediterranean diet to menopausal women who have experienced weight gain. I don't do diets, nor do I write about them, and I'm heartened that our culture is finally recognizing that for the vast majority of people, diets don't work. But the Mediterranean diet is less a dreary "diet" than a plant-based healthy eating plan. It was introduced in the 1950s when it was noted that people in Mediterranean countries like Greece had longer life spans and lower rates of heart disease. Beloved by nutritionists, it's characterized by foods with antioxidant and anti-inflammatory properties, includes vegetables, fruits, "good" fats like extra-virgin olive oil, nuts, red wine, and whole-grain cereals. "Several evidences showed that the Mediterranean diet acts on both weight control and menopause," the researchers write.

Not only that, says Dr. Pauline Maki at the University of Illinois at Chicago, "there's actually really good data to show that the Mediterranean diet lowers the risk of preclinical Alzheimer's disease. Imagine that—a diet, in a very large, randomized trial, was shown to decrease the risk of this type of dementia that we're all afraid of."

This doesn't mean you have to adhere to the Mediterranean diet all day long, Maki adds. You can do things like substitute butter for olive oil or swap out your snack foods for hummus and carrots.

And no, specific foods can't "balance" your hormones, no matter what claims people make on social media or in various cookbooks. As ob-gyn Jen Gunter, author of *The Menopause Manifesto*, wrote in *The New York Times*, the idea that reproductive hormones need to be "in balance" is "a common modern myth in gynecology exam rooms all across North America." A woman's hormone levels, she reminds us, "change not only day to day, but also often hour to hour." Therefore they cannot be "balanced."

It's worth cutting back on salt, too. As mentioned earlier, a decline in estrogen after menopause increases your risk of developing high blood pressure; using less salt may lower that risk. Salt is not good for your bones, either: a 2018 Korean study found an association between high dietary sodium intake and low bone mass in postmenopausal women. The American Heart Association recommends 1,500 milligrams or less per day (although this guideline may not apply to people who sweat a lot, so if you happen to be a competitive athlete, foundry worker, or firefighter, the AHA says you may need more).

• • • •

A few days after I phone my sisters about their hair, Heather calls me. "Okay, this is weird," she says. "I was just looking at the skin on the back of my right hand, and it has this strange pattern on it."

I put the kettle on; might as well settle in for this. "What sort of pattern?"

"It looks like this sort of hexagonal print is on my hand. Like I've been leaning on a pillow or something, and it made a mark. But I don't have any pillows, or anything else, really, that would make a hexagonal print. It's not on my bedspread or anything. It's not like I've been, you know, leaning on a honeycomb. What could it be?"

I am mystified. I tell her to wait fifteen minutes, see if the honeycomb disappears, and then call me back. In the meantime, I google "honeycomb hands" and wish I hadn't; it takes me to an obscure skin condition with extremely disturbing pictures.

I have just finished my tea when Heather calls me back. "It's still there," she says. "It's still there on the back of my hand."

"Which hand?" I ask, even as I wonder why on earth this is relevant. She tells me it's her left.

"What about your other hand?"

"I've just decided not to look at my hands anymore," she says. She pauses for a minute. "Now you made me look, and the right hand is honeycombed, too. Shit."

“Let me investigate.” I tell her to text me a picture.

“Honestly, now that I’m really looking at it, it doesn’t bother me all that much,” Heather says. “I’m already sort of accepting it. It is what it is.”

“But maybe it isn’t what it is,” I say, refilling my mug of tea.

“You want to know something twisted?” Heather asks.

Who would say no to that? Not I.

“Remember when Dad got his knee replacement surgery last month? Well, he showed me his leg, and it was so swollen that there wasn’t one wrinkle or dip. And I was jealous! I said, ‘Dad, don’t you love your leg? It’s like a toddler’s leg.’”

“I’m looking at the picture, okay? You do not have honeycomb hands. Your skin is just dry.”

While I did not notice honeycomb patterns on my own body, the most dramatic change in my appearance during menopause was undoubtedly my skin. Over a few years, it transformed from decently supple to parched, irritable, zit-covered, and slack.

Estrogen plays a role in the production of collagen, a major structural protein in skin that helps to maintain firmness, elasticity, and hydration levels, and even aids in wound healing. An estimated 30 percent of dermal collagen may be lost in the first five years after menopause; after that, collagen continues to tick downward at about 2 percent per year, while thickness declines by about 1 percent a year. “If it makes you feel any better,” says Corey L. Hartman, assistant clinical professor of dermatology at the University of Alabama School of Medicine, “everybody’s losing collagen all the time.”

Loss of estrogen, and the subsequent depletion of collagen, can make skin prone to thinning, dryness, sensitivity, and dullness. “Our skin loses its firmness and begins to sag,” reports the website of the American Academy of Dermatology. “Jowls appear. Permanent lines run from the tip of the nose to the corner of the mouth. Wrinkles that used to appear only with a smile or frown become visible all the time." Finally, this: "Later, *the tip of the nose dips* [italics mine]."

During perimenopause and menopause, you may be blessed with both acne and wrinkles, as I was when zits gathered in the ever-deepening creases on either side of my mouth (dismayingly called "parentheses" or "marionette lines" by plastic surgeons).

At around the age of fifty, the pH level of our skin changes, according to the AAD. As this pH level climbs, those cells are less able to help defend the skin. With this change, skin becomes weaker and more sensitive. If you have an existing skin condition like rosacea or eczema, it could worsen.

Not only does collagen drop with age, so do levels of elastin, another protein that, true to its name, gives skin its resilience and bounce. Your complexion can look pulled down (sometimes known as Resting Bitch Face). I developed jowls and a dewlap—that would be a longitudinal flap of skin that hangs beneath the lower jaw of many vertebrates. I found my own Resting Bitch Face particularly upsetting because I suddenly looked dour, which didn't at all match my internal energy and optimism.

I share this inner joie de vivre with my mother. Mom is a former Alabama beauty pageant queen who is . . . I was about to write that she is "still lovely at eighty," but then I remembered the model Paulina Porizkova's denouncement of the word *still.*

Porizkova, born in 1965, is a delightfully vocal opponent of how dismissive our society is to women as they age. She exhorts women to stand up and insist on not being invisible. On her Instagram account, she called out men who regularly message her that she's "still" beautiful, she's "still" hot, they'd "still" date her. "Can we please do away with the 'still'?!" she writes of these blatantly ageist remarks. "A 'still' is like a 'but.' One ruins a compliment, the other ruins an apology. The word 'still' in this connotes your surprise at someone 'still' being what your assumption of them was. Which in this case is what? No longer beautiful? How many times do you hear, 'You're still smart. You're still talented.' Not often, right?

"The next time you're tempted to insert a 'still,'" concludes Porizkova, "take a moment, and don't."

She is right. Ageism, especially when paired with sexism, is insidious and relentless. Even as I face ageism myself, I am sometimes unaware of how I've internalized it—how it has crept into my perceptions and language, which I am trying to check.

While Porizkova's point is that women should not be scorned for, as she has often put it, daring to age, I am not quite there yet (which she has maintained she understands, too). I want my face to reflect the vibrancy that I feel inside. Like my friend Kathy, I have more energy now than I did when I was in my constantly hungover twenties.

I have written about skin for many years for *Vogue* and have interviewed countless dermatologists. I enlist their help to craft an action plan.

First, get ready to overhaul your skin routine, says Dr. Corey L. Hartman. I tell Hartman that when I entered perimenopause, all of my go-to products, such as moisturizer, sat uselessly on the top of my skin. During perimenopause, cell turnover slows—and my skin had formed a dry, hardened layer that nothing was penetrating. "One of the biggest mistakes people make is using the same thing throughout their lives," he says. When menopause hits, he says, "patients will say to me, 'I don't understand it, I haven't changed anything.' Well, that's part of the problem."

I then visit Shereene Idriss, a clinical instructor in dermatology at the Icahn School of Medicine at Mount Sinai, at Idriss Dermatology,

“After menopause, your hormones change, your shape changes. Your belly gets bigger, too. I’m constantly having to work on loving that part of my body. It’s so hard. If I ever say anything demeaning about myself, because I’ve taught [my daughters] not to do that, they’ll say, ‘Why are you doing what you told us not to do?’ Aging is a really, really intimate educator on loving yourself, because you can’t stop it. It’s going to happen.”

—Andie MacDowell

which overlooks leafy Bryant Park in New York City. Her namesake office reflects the exuberant personality that has made Idriss a social media star. Color-coded gumballs and chocolate bonbons are piled in glass jars in the waiting room; Dr. Idriss's own artwork and a neon sign reading WEAR THE DAMN SUNSCREEN adorn the walls. An olive tree is a nod to her Lebanese heritage.

She rolls into the office, hair caught in a shiny ponytail, her fatigue pants and gold sneakers peeking out from under her crisp white coat, and launches into a tutorial on menopausal skin. Along with collagen production, she tells me as she paces the room, waning estrogen levels also deplete your body's store of ceramides, fatty acids that are essential to keeping skin cells intact and help to maintain the skin barrier and retain hydration. Levels of hyaluronic acid—a molecule that gives your dermis structure and squishy bounce—also dip.

How, then, do we restore moisture and springiness?

Bid adieu to harsh soaps. "They can further dry out our skin and further break up our skin barrier," says Idriss. "Instead, we want to use creamy, rich cleansers." Avoid heavily fragranced products, too, and take warm, not hot showers, which strip your skin of natural oils. For gentle cleansing of the body, Idriss and many other derms love Cetaphil cleansers; she also recommends Aveeno Nourishing Oat Cleanser, which is fragrance-free. Dove Sensitive Skin Beauty Bar gets high marks from doctors, such as New York City dermatologist Joshua Zeichner.

Add retinols to your skin-care routine. This is the time to seek out biologically active ingredients for your skincare, rather than ones that just moisturize. Put your products to work! If you didn't start using retinol earlier in life, it's never too late. Retinol, the vitamin A derivative, revs cell renewal (which brightens skin and fades sunspots) and helps your skin boost its own collagen production.

"Retinol is obviously a great one, but the problem is that in perimenopausal women, our collagen stores are already sort of depleted, so retinols can be irritating," says Idriss. If you are new to retinols, start slowly. Apply twice a week at night, followed by moisturizer. And look for products with soothing ingredients such as glycerin. "If you find retinol is still too irritating," says Idriss, "go for creams that are loaded in peptides."

Several derms recommend L'Oréal's Revitalift Night Serum with Pure Retinol, while NYC derm Macrene Alexiades favors RoC Retinol Correxion Line Smoothing Eye Cream. Many derms are fans of the Ordinary's Granactive Retinoid 2% in Squalene and CeraVe's Skin Renewing Retinol Serum; both are good for sensitive skin.

If your skin can handle it, Dr. Alexiades recommends tretinoin, a stronger version of retinol available by prescription. "When you stop ovulating, the skin isn't boosted every month with a nice vascular nutrient-rich skin layer, there are fewer nutrients to the skin, and the epidermis starts to thin," says the eminent dermatologist with three Harvard degrees when I visit her in her elegant office on New York City's Upper East Side. "I put in place ingredients that will substitute for the lack of estrogenic effect, and if you don't have sensitive skin, retinoids stimulate the production of new blood vessels in the skin."

Fortify your skin barrier. The outermost part of the epidermis, your skin barrier keeps moisture in and environmental threats out. Strengthen it with a moisturizer that has ingredients like the ceramides that Dr. Idriss mentioned. Research shows that melanin-rich skin has lower levels of ceramides, so darker skin during menopause can be more prone to dryness and ashiness.

For ceramides, two products have come up again and again from the dermatologists I've consulted over the years: Aveeno Skin Relief Intense Moisture Repair Cream and CeraVe Moisturizing Cream.

Misting is your friend. Drenching your skin with mist, says Idriss, is good for both hydrating and the occasional hot flash. "But misting just with water might dehydrate your skin, counterintuitively, if water is just sitting on the surface," Idriss says, pausing this delightful private tutorial to open a cabinet piled full of Milano cookies and offer me a pack. "Mix water with a little bit of glycerin and even some rose water to help with inflammation and put it in a misting bottle or a mister that you can buy on Amazon. This is a great thing to keep in your purse or on your desk at work and to use a couple of times throughout the day." Heritage Store Rosewater & Glycerin Hydrating Facial Mist is inexpensive, smells delicious, moisturizes, and tamps my nighttime hot flashes. It never leaves my bedside table.

Treat the skin on your body with extra care. Your skin everywhere has become thinner, more fragile, and in need of nourishment, so "treat the skin on your body with caution, almost like you're an eczema patient," says Idriss. (In fact, for guaranteed gentleness, look for products emblazoned with a seal of approval from the National Eczema Association.) "And make sure you're moisturizing with a really thick, rich ointment." Idriss favors Aquaphor Advanced Therapy Ointment Body Spray ("it dries relatively fast without leaving any residual tackiness"), while New York City dermatologist Dr. Blair Murphy-Rose likes Curél Ultra Healing Lotion.

For the body, several derms also recommend virgin or extra-virgin coconut oil. (This has been cold-pressed from fresh coconut meat, rather than conventional coconut oil, which is more processed and made from dried coconut meat.) It's rich in beneficial fatty acids like lauric acid, which is antibacterial and can protect fragile skin, and intensely hydrating linoleic acid. I tried it, and now it's a staple in my bathroom—it's nourishing, penetrates my skin, is delicately fragrant, and adds luster by subtly reflecting light.

Costco makes an enormous 84-ounce vat of organic cold-pressed virgin coconut oil that costs under twenty bucks and last for ages.

Build lost collagen with peptides. Peptides, which are short-chain amino acids that are absorbed by the skin, improve tone, texture, and firmness. "They boost collagen and elastin and are generally non-irritating," says Alexiades. She recommends Olay Regenerist Collagen Peptide 24 Hydrating Moisturizer; I join the chorus of derms who love CeraVe's peptide-rich Skin Renewing Night Cream. Nothing penetrated my lizard-like outer-skin layer and restored my complexion more effectively, and you can get it at the drugstore.

Boost moisture with hyaluronic acid. Hyaluronic acid, which is naturally produced by our bodies, can hold a thousand times its weight in water. It's an ideal way, says Alexiades, to replenish moisture and reduce lines. Don't be thrown by the word *acid*—it's a healing ingredient that's been shown, in higher doses, to speed wound healing. Paula's Choice Skin Recovery Replenishing Moisturizer and the Ordinary Hyaluronic Acid 2% are often mentioned by the dermatologists I interview.

Your menopausal acne may linger for a while, so treat it. Many women report an outbreak of acne on their newly dry skin, especially around their chin (like me) and jawline. While oil production decreases during the menopause transition, Dr. Hartman explains, "the instability of the hormones can cause acne to flare up, which seems like an awful irony when oil is usually the thing that causes the acne to flare in the first place."

Treat breakouts with care, Hartman says. Put down your teen's zit cream, for starters. "All acne is not created the same," he says. "Teenage skin has lots of oil and can easily tolerate some of these harsh products, but women going through menopause will have side effects."

Because menopausal acne is driven by hormonal changes, Hartman recommends a prescription cream called clascoterone (Winlevi is the product name), which targets specific acne-causing hormones in the skin, while Alexiades recommends clearing acne from the inside out with an oral dose of spironolactone. It slows down your body's production of androgen hormones, she says, which make the skin produce too much oil. (And if you happen to have the double delight of acne and hair loss, spironolactone, as previously noted, treats that, too.)

Look for acne products specifically formulated for sensitive skin, such as La Roche-Posay's Effaclar Duo Dual Action Acne Treatment Cream, which uses gentle beta-lipohydroxy acid to unclog pores, is fragrance-free, and is fortified with skin-calming glycerin.

And yes, wear the damn sunscreen. Over the years, I have talked to well over a hundred dermatologists, and overwhelmingly, they agree that if an actual fountain of youth existed, sunscreen would be spouting out of it.

It's easily the best method to keep skin plump and fresh. UV radiation from the sun directly breaks down the collagen in your skin, so use a 30 to 50 SPF, says Idriss, every day—yes, in winter, yes on cloudy days, and yes, darker skins need daily sunblock. "Every single human being needs to apply sunscreen, regardless of their skin tone."

"It's never too late to join the sunscreen bandwagon," says Idriss. handing me another pack of Milano cookies, which I rip open and eat right in the treatment room. "Protect the skin you have and start loading up." Dermatologist-vetted sunscreens for menopausal skin include Eucerin Sun Face Cream Sensitive Protect 50+, Neutrogena Sensitive Skin Face 50, and Black Girl Make It Matte Broad Spectrum SPF 45.

And if you want to make a menopausal woman's day, just give

her an enormous container of Costco virgin coconut oil. After my conversation with Heather, we met up for soup dumplings at a restaurant we love that's in between our hometowns. "I have a surprise for you," I announce in a singsong voice when we meet in the parking lot, and heave it into the back seat of her car.

She calls me the next day. "No more honeycomb hands," she says jubilantly.

Chapter 7

Why Did I Walk Into This Room Again?

Brain Fog Is Real. So Are Mood Changes.

I'm buying groceries at Stop & Shop, where I seem to spend half my waking hours, when a woman with brown hair runs up to me in Cleaning Supplies and Paper Goods.

"Jancee!" she cries. "How are you?"

I have no idea who this person is. I paste a smile on my face.

"Hey, you!" I say brightly. The phrase *Hey, you* fools absolutely no one, but it's all I've got at the moment.

"Oh my god, Jancee, it's been forever! How's Tom?" she asks. *Shit, she knows my husband's name?*

"He's great," I say, nodding too quickly. *Who the hell* are *you? Are you a parent at my kid's school? My cat sitter? Wait, are you my dentist? Usually you have that visor thing covering your face.*

She stares at me expectantly. "How's the family?" I ask finally. *Everyone has some sort of family, right?*

As the mystery woman gives me some family news about one of her kids who is off to college, I do a mind trick I've been relying on more and more often: I go through the alphabet, hoping it will shake loose some sort of memory of her name. A . . . Alia? Amanda?

The downside of having an unusual moniker like mine is that people tend to remember it. I was born pre-sonogram, and my parents confidently, and sort of weirdly, assumed I'd be a boy—so much so that they didn't bother picking a girl's name. I was to be the third J.C. in my family, after James Curtis, the name of my dad and grandfather. When they discovered I was a girl, they made up the name Jancee on the spot.

As mentioned earlier, Dad—and my granddad—worked their entire lives for the JCPenney company, so the name J.C. has mystical powers in the Dunn household. My grandfather even hosted James Cash Penney himself (yes, his real name) for lunch at his home. A photo of the momentous event, the equivalent of a priest in some obscure parish being visited by the Pope, hung in our living room for years, near a stately bronze bust of J. C. Penney's head. I have a cousin named Penny, too—guess where she worked?

The Stop & Shop woman is still talking. I am up to M in the alphabet when I finally hit upon it: Mara. My neighbor down the street.

"Great to see you, Mara!" I chirp as I head for the checkout line.

• • • •

My mental fumbling, research shows, is familiar to many. Nearly a quarter of women in menopause experience changes in brain function, according to a 2022 review in *Best Practice & Research Clinical Obstetrics & Gynaecology*. Other large-scale studies of my menopausal comrades find consistent changes in memory, verbal learning, and processing speed.

"I would get so low, really, really low, beaten, like never before. It just came out of nowhere. I'm like, 'Well, you are pushing fifty, girl. At some point things are going to change.' I still have to manage it. That means talking to my therapist when I feel this way, [like] doing things to get me out of the muck."

—Tariji P. Henson

While this may be commonplace, it's still, to say the least, alarming. "Very often," says Wen Shen of Johns Hopkins, "a patient will come in and tell me that she thinks she's losing her mind."

Estrogen stimulates neural activity in the brain—so when it wanes, the brain is affected. "Menopausal symptoms such as depression and hot flashes arise from biological changes in your brain, which people don't recognize," says Hadine Joffe of Harvard. "They think it's in the ovaries. I always tell people that the brain is really at the helm here, and all these hormones have effects on all kinds of things, like cognition, mood, and migraines."

Researchers didn't actually know until the 1990s, Joffe says, that female hormones such as estrogen and progesterone, and male hormones such as testosterone, "are active in the brain, outside of the reproductive centers." Both men and women have estrogen receptors, and men—who knew?—have receptors in their penises as well as their brains.

When I talk to Pauline Maki at the University of Illinois at Chicago, I feel an enormous sense of relief. She confirms that I'm not imagining my brain fog—and that it's likely not going to last. "Brain fog and memory problems are a normal experience through menopause," says Maki, whose work focuses on the effects of sex hormones on cognition, brain function, and psychological well-being in women. "It's normal, it's measurable, and we see this in our studies routinely."

Maki, who has followed large groups of women through the menopause transition, has observed a discernible change in their cognitive performance on certain tests. Although not everyone gets brain fog, she hastens to add. "Some people sail through menopause with nary a problem. There are different levels of hormone sensitivity, and I think that applies to cognition as well." But for those of us who have an inability to remember and concentrate, Maki says, it seems to begin as soon as a woman's menstrual cycle starts to become irregular in perimenopause.

I tell her that when I can't remember names like Mara's or walk into a room and forget why I'm there, I'm frequently afraid that Alzheimer's disease is coming for me. I know that women are disproportionately affected by Alzheimer's; for reasons that are still unclear, nearly two-thirds of Americans with the disease, according to the Alzheimer's Association, are female. "Right," Maki says. "That's a very common fear. And as somebody whose grandmother passed away with Alzheimer's disease, this is a huge concern for me, too."

The good news, she says, is that for the "very, very large majority of women, this has nothing to do with Alzheimer's disease." That affliction, she adds, is in fact very rare in midlife. Note: If you forget where you've put your keys, doctors say, you're normal. If you don't know what the keys are *for*, you might have a problem.

Maki says that one compelling reason why this memory loss isn't necessarily dire is that "longitudinal studies have shown that memory bounces back in postmenopause—that in general it's this time-limited thing," says Maki. "We have very good data to suggest that. So if this is setting you up on a different course for Alzheimer's disease, why would memory bounce back?"

Neuroscientist Lisa Mosconi, who directs Weill Cornell Women's Brain Initiative, also studies how menopause refashions the landscape of the female brain. She has said that we should look at the brain as something that's impacted by menopause at least as much as our ovaries are.

In a 2021 study published in the journal *Scientific Reports*, Mosconi and her colleagues examined the brains of women at different stages of menopause (pre-, peri-, and post-) to investigate its effects on the brain's gray matter (the cells that process information) and white matter, the fibers that connect those cells. They found that the women experienced a drop in the brain's gray matter volume in a region called the precuneus, believed to be involved in memory and social cognition. White matter also decreased, along with the brain's consumption of glucose, the main fuel source for cells.

But women's resourceful brains at least partly compensated for these declines by boosting blood flow and producing a molecule called ATP, another energy source for cells. In effect, their brains were remodeling themselves without estrogen. Follow-up scans on the women two years after menopause found that cognitive changes not only seemed temporary, but typically reversed themselves a few years after the women reached menopause.

In other words, you will not always call butter *the yellow stuff that you spread on bread. Hold on, give me a minute. It's on the tip of my tongue. You spread it with a shiny silver thing.* As Dr. Mosconi put it, the study suggested "that the brain has an ability to find a new 'normal' after menopause, at least in most women."

While the mental muddiness does pass for most of us, those with hot flashes and night sweats and the resulting poor sleep, says Maki, might not bounce back. Her research has found a link between how many hot flashes a woman has and her memory performance. "That chronic sleep deprivation, night after night, can contribute directly and indirectly to memory problems," says Maki. "For some women, these hot flashes continue for up to a decade or more, particularly in women of color."

That's why it's so important, as we've said throughout these pages, to treat severe hot flashes if they interfere with your sleep. More rest should improve your memory, Maki says.

I'm comforted to know my vagueness will, hopefully, pass, and my memory will likely come back. How many physiological functions return after they're gone? It's a small miracle.

Sometimes my memory blanks out for longer than a minute. During a trip to the mall, I forgot where I left my car in the parking garage. I wandered around for an hour, too embarrassed to ask the mall security guy to help me find it—or maybe I didn't want to be perceived as helpless. When I finally found my car, I was fighting back tears. (Pro tip: Take a picture of the car park number with your phone.)

• • • •

Depression and mood changes during menopause have been chronicled since the nineteenth century. In his 1857 book on menopause, *The Change of Life in Health and Disease,* physician and author Dr. Edward Tilt wrote about menopausal women's "unusual peevishness and ill-temper, sometimes assuming the importance of moral insanity. Some make their once-peaceful homes intolerable by their ungovernable temper; others bear hatred, for a time, to the long-cherished objects of their affection."

The good doctor nailed the hatred for "long-cherished objects of affection" part; he was less prescient with his gargantuan list of the 120 symptoms of menopause, which make our 34 seem trifling. They include "boils in seat," "obstinate constipation," "hysterical paralysis of arms," "fainting away repeatedly," "bleeding piles," "falling off of all the nails," and a mysterious but ghastly seeming condition called "pus in motions."

Fortunately, Dr. Tilt had a profusion of remedies in his arsenal, among them opium, morphine, belladonna, and lead acetate, a toxic compound now used in insecticides, as a coating for metals, and a drying agent in varnishes. Dr. Tilt injected lead acetate directly into women's vaginas—perhaps not the best place for industrial-grade drying agents and a "cure" that probably caused the women to "faint away repeatedly" if they weren't doing it already.

A towering pile of research shows a link between women's ping-ponging hormones and mood. As mentioned earlier, women are already nearly twice as likely as men to experience major depression; hormones can toss another wrench into the proceedings.

There are three main hormonally linked mood conditions in women, according to Hadine Joffe at Harvard University. They are postpartum depression (PPD), premenstrual syndrome (PMS), and perimenopausal depression. Thankfully, you can't experience all three at once. (Or can you? I contact Dr. Minkin at Yale Medical School to double check. "It's unlikely that a postpartum woman will be perimenopausal," she says, "but of course it's possible, if, let's say, she had donor eggs.")

The same hormones that control your menstrual cycle also have an effect on serotonin, which is a neurotransmitter, or chemical messenger, in the brain that promotes those delicious feelings of contentment and happiness. When hormone levels drop, so, too, do serotonin levels. The resulting feelings of irritability and ready anger call up author Sandra Tsing Loh's description of menopause in *The Atlantic,* where "a woman can feel like the only way she can continue to exist for ten more seconds inside her crawling, burning skin is to walk screaming into the sea—grandly, epically, and terrifyingly."

For some people entering the menopause transition, levels of depression and anxiety may spike—again, particularly, several large studies show, if they have had a previous diagnosis of depression or anxiety disorder. "The majority of women who have a history of depression will in fact experience a recurrence of their depression during the menopausal transition," says Maki. "We're beginning to understand why this is the case, and to appreciate that some women's biological response to stress is strongly linked to hormone fluctuations." If this is part of your medical history, Maki adds, let your doctor know.

Perimenopause seems to be an especially susceptible time for depression. A 2011 SWAN study found that women were two to four times more likely to experience a major depressive episode (MDE) when they were perimenopausal.

Because the physical symptoms of menopause can be so intense and pervasive, it's often easy to overlook the mental symptoms. But the risk of depression is elevated in perimenopause even among women with *no* history of depression. If emotional ups and downs during perimenopause or menopause are getting in the way of functioning everyday life, see your doctor. In fact, experts say that women should be routinely screened for depression in perimenopause, which is now seen as a "window of vulnerability," not unlike the postpartum period, for depressive symptoms to creep in.

Dr. Minkin says she has found that for perimenopausal depression, a low-dose birth control pill called Yaz can be helpful for patients. Yaz is FDA-approved to treat premenstrual dysphoric disorder (PMDD), a more severe form of PMS—including symptoms of depression and anxiety.

Because women in midlife are often knee-deep in major issues—aging parents, needy teens, job worries, health scares, divorce, money paranoia—it can be hard to separate a depressive episode or anxiety disorder from general life stress.

The classic signs of an anxiety disorder may be worries that you can't seem to turn off, persistent feelings of doom, panic attacks, and a racing heart.

Depression, meanwhile, can feel like a sadness you are unable to escape, or profound and incessant feelings of hopelessness and emptiness. It can manifest as a loss of interest in activities that used to make you happy, eating or sleeping more or less than usual, or a lack of energy that flattens you so thoroughly that even small tasks take effort. If you experience these sorts of symptoms nearly every day for two or more weeks, see your doctor.

And be forthright with your doctor about your mental health symptoms, says Joffe. "If you have a rash, you'd get it treated, right?" she says. "This is no different."

• • • •

I have not had major depression, but mood swings are a different story. At a store called Tons of Toys that my daughter liked to visit, I began to avoid a certain shelf filled with stuffed animals, because they all looked so sadly hopeful to me—like Corduroy, the little bear in the children's book, who waited patiently day after day with the other animals and dolls for someone to take him home. I couldn't look at these inanimate objects without getting a hitch in my throat. I found their sweet smiles unbearable. I wanted to take them all.

And anger boiled up out of nowhere, such as the time I screamed, "Fuck you!" at *my pants* when I couldn't button them up. My friend Shira relays a similar story. She was checking out at a crowded bodega, her arms full of groceries, when a man suddenly stepped in front of her and tried to get the cashier to stop serving her and ring up his single banana first. "It's just a quick sale," he kept insisting.

"Normally, I just would have shrugged and let him jump in front of me," she says. "But something about his entitlement, his rudeness, and his utter lack of disregard for bodega norms sparked a rage in me. This man was every man who had ever tried to cut in line in front of me over the last forty years. For the first time, I understood the meaning of the phrase *seeing red*—I was so outrageously, self-righteously, incandescently mad in that moment."

A heated shouting match erupted. "I eventually left the store with my stuff, vibrating with anger after having made a scene," she says. "It was totally unlike me. About two blocks later, as the adrenaline left my body and my heart rate slowed, I started marveling at this fury that I'd felt rushing through me. This menopausal madness scared me a little, but part of me was also fascinated by it."

Another normally chill friend went into an uncharacteristic tirade at her husband for leaving several layers of dishes in the sink. She hollered at him and then dramatically smashed his favorite mug on the floor, where it broke into pieces. When she saw his crestfallen face, she burst into hysterical tears.

To be fair to her, the battle over dishwashing can be especially fraught in relationships—to the point where one manufacturer announced plans to make an "argument-proof" appliance. Research published in 2018 in *Socius*, a journal of the American Sociological Association, found that how couples divvy up dishwashing duty can be a litmus test of their relationship. It can even drag down your sex life. Dan Carlson, an associate professor of family and consumer studies at the University of Utah, studied the domestic habits of low- to moderate-income parents who shared routine household tasks like shopping, laundry, cooking, and cleaning. He and his colleagues found that among the women in the study, those who found themselves doing most of the dishwashing "reported significantly more relationship discord, lower relationship satisfaction, and less sexual satisfaction than women who split the dishes with their partner," Carlson wrote. Lack of sharing of dishwashing in particular was "the biggest source of discontent."

I decided to compare stories of menopausal mood at one of my

"I suffered brain fog and anxiety to the extent I thought I was losing my mind. I thought, 'I'm not okay, I think I got a brain tumor, or Alzheimer's or something.'"

—English TV presenter Davina McCall

extended family's many gatherings. We all readily show up and eat together on the flimsiest of pretenses. On this particular day, we were celebrating that my father's left leg had healed up nicely from his knee replacement operation (the one that had sparked envy from Heather). If I had been more prepared, I would have brought a festive knee-shaped cake.

On a rainy winter Sunday, my whole family—parents; two younger sisters, Dinah and Heather; various nieces and nephews; and my kid—is crammed in Heather's kitchen, despite having other perfectly good rooms to catch the spillover. We always do this; it's probably because the kitchen has all the food.

As we gather around an enormous bowl of pico de gallo, brandishing chips, I ask my mom and sisters about menopausal mood swings, and share that I had recently yelled at my pants that had stubbornly refused to close over the canned biscuit dough of my stomach.

My husband, Tom, looks uncomfortable as he heaves a vast basin of guacamole onto the table. I hold his gaze, daring him to walk away. *Oh, no you don't,* I inform him telepathically. *We are all going to move the societal needle and speak freely and casually about this normal life stage, here and now!* He loads a chip with guac and reluctantly sits on a stool.

Dinah reaches for a chip. "I don't know if I had mood issues, but I had lost my job and was starting a divorce when I began perimenopause, so it's hard to tell," she says. "It's hard to separate it all, because it's a time in your life where there's a lot going on."

"Mood-wise, I had feelings of being overwhelmed," Heather chimes in. "Then again, so much was going on with me, too." When her perimenopausal symptoms cranked up, she had just started a job as a special education teacher.

Dinah nods. "I did feel really sad that I could never have kids again. I wasn't planning on it, but to have that choice taken away from me was a little depressing. I was done. You know? If I'd had a different life, I probably would have had more kids."

This is the first I've heard that she had wanted more children. I run over and give her a hug.

"You know what?" says Dinah. "It's not all bad. The transition of going into menopause was like a turning point for me. It felt like a starter pistol, in a way. In my marriage, I was like, 'I'm done, our daughters are older, I don't have much time left. And I don't need to deal with you anymore.' I got divorced. I started my own book company. I began going out again with my friends and trying new things. And I realized I was more self-sufficient than I thought."

My mom narrows her eyes. "I remember my moods would go up and down—mostly down. I would get really mean." She jumps up and refills her glass of wine. "When that happened, your father would find another place to be, because I was a ring-tailed bitch."

I glance at my dad, who is clearly weighing whether to confirm or deny, finally deciding, like some Kofi Annan of the suburban kitchen, it is perhaps best to do neither.

"Everything he did just bugged the shit out of me," Mom goes on. "God, I hated your father!" She glares at him, remembering. "Hated, hated, hated," she continues in a chillingly singsong voice.

Dad pretends to be deeply absorbed in his corn chips.

• • • •

Falling estrogen and progesterone levels can indeed trigger a flurry of different moods.

These touchy, reactive feelings—kind of like having PMS all the time—are also not in your imagination, says Maki. "Research has shown that if you follow large numbers of women as they transition through menopause, there are reports of depressive symptoms, so it's validated," she says. "It doesn't meet the clinical criteria for depression, but nevertheless does affect our well-being. We just don't feel as engaged, we feel a little more blue, we're not as interested in the activities that we typically like. And really, the most helpful thing we doctors can do is normalize these experiences and let women know that their brains really are sensitive to fluctuating levels of estrogen, both in terms of cognitive ability and mood."

As with memory problems, Maki wants to be clear that many women ably roll into menopause without serious mental health issues. "Again, many women sail through and are fine," she says. "However, it can be a very different experience for women with a history of mental health difficulties." Talk therapy and cognitive behavioral therapy have been shown to be helpful for mood swings, too, says Joffe.

Therapy, I know, is not cheap. If your insurance does not cover it, the Open Path Psychotherapy Collective—see Resources—is a nonprofit nationwide network of mental health professionals who provide in-office mental health care at a steeply reduced rate, starting at $30 per session. Similarly, *Psychology Today*'s website features a "find a therapist" service to locate a counselor near you, and you can set the price.

Some therapists will accept sliding-scale fees based on a client's ability to pay. Many colleges and universities with mental health practitioner programs offer sessions with counselors in training that are open to the public, often with affordable sliding-scale fees. I've had excellent sessions with grad students in training who were just as diligent as longtime therapists. Low-fee clinics are another option. The American Psychoanalytic Association has a list of low-fee clinics across the country. If you're an active member of the military, YMCA memberships are free for you and your family—and a little-known fact is that many branches of the Y offer mental health counseling for members.

Support groups are free and can be tremendously helpful. Facebook groups like Perimenopause WTF?!, which counts over 11,000 members ("Your Perimenopause Sisterhood"), overflows with empathy and I've-been-there advice. No matter what kooky experience you've been through, someone else will have gone through it as well and will comment with a reassuring *Girl, me too.* ("I have spent the entire day crying, but absolutely nothing is bothering me." "I can't remember my dogs' names." "My head feels like it's full of rocks sometimes and there's only tiny gaps where I can take stuff in.")

Finally, be mindful that, as mentioned repeatedly throughout this book, menopausal sleep loss can have a direct impact on depression and mood swings. NAMS does *not* recommend menopausal hormone therapy at any age to prevent or treat a decline in cognitive function, although it gives MHT thumbs-up for treating hot flashes and sleep disturbances, which might have a positive effect on memory and concentration.

"If people are having nighttime hot flashes that are interrupting their sleep, we see the effect on mood," says Joffe, who stresses that it's "hugely important" to protect your sleep as part of protecting mood. "We don't prioritize sleep," she says. "It's something we feel is flexible, as opposed to, 'No, I need to prioritize it, this is my health.'" (This is where some antidepressants that have been shown to ease physical symptoms of menopause may also help.)

Every expert I talked to said to bolster your mental health with the usual suspects: eat well, try to keep your stress down, and get regular exercise.

At this point, we all know that exercise is good for mental

"You have the hormonal shifts, you're not quite sure who you are anymore, what you're supposed to become, and I basically was having a nervous breakdown. I couldn't speak above a whisper. I couldn't eat. I had to walk very slowly. I had to listen to very soft, soothing music. I was very, very, very vulnerable."

—Jane Fonda

well-being. A meta-analysis of twenty-five randomized clinical trials concluded that exercise has a large and significant antidepressant effect among people diagnosed with major depressive disorder.

But the reality is that a workout can be tough to fit in. I've been a little better about my exercise regimen since I rebranded it in my mind as *movement,* after reading Dr. Kelly McGonigal's *The Joy of Movement*. The Stanford University lecturer's message is that physical activity contributes to human happiness. She says to consider every time you get up and move your body purposefully and joyfully as a win. "Our entire physiology was designed to reward us for moving," she writes. "If you are willing to move, your brain will orchestrate pleasure."

McGonigal advises that you not think of exercise as a grim pursuit to burn calories or hit some gym-circuitry milestone. Instead she suggests that you start with a set of simple questions: What brings you joy? What movement did you love as a child? What movement would you do just for the sheer fun of it, even if it didn't yield results? And, she asks further, can you pair movement with things that already bring you joy? It's one of the oldest motivational tricks, but it works: Create some enthusiasm for something you *don't* want to do by pairing it with something you're excited to do.

This method, known as temptation bundling, was described in a 2014 study published in the journal *Management Science*. Temptation bundling pairs instantly gratifying *wants*, like checking social media or watching some nice, junky reality TV, with *shoulds*, like doing your taxes, which "provide long-term benefits but require the exertion of willpower." In the study, subjects given an iPod loaded with audiobooks that they could listen to only at the gym worked out 51 percent more than those with no iPod. It fired up the subjects so much that after the study ended, three-fifths of them said that they would pay their own money for gym-only audiobooks.

Can you phone a friend you adore and haven't talked to in a while and chat as you walk? If music lights you up, maybe you can walk while catching up with New Music Friday on Spotify? (A 2022 study published in the journal *Menopause* found that menopausal women who listened to music as a form of therapy had a "significant decrease" in depressive symptoms.)

I take a page from the study and do a little self-bribery, allowing myself to listen to my beloved true-crime podcasts only if I take an hour-long fast walk. Each podcast inevitably ends in a cliffhanger, so I can hardly wait to get out there and move again, if only to find out if the murderer was the creepy neighbor or the unconvincingly mild-mannered choir director.

I also joined my local YMCA so that I could swim, an activity I loved as a kid. As it happens, it's the very Y where I took swimming lessons growing up. After living in Brooklyn for twenty years, I recently moved to my home state of New Jersey to be near my family—and found a house that was a mere five-minute drive from my hometown, an experience that has been slightly surreal. One afternoon, on the way to the Y to swim, I grabbed an old Reagan-era jean jacket of mine that my parents had excavated from their attic during one of their periodic purges. (As my mother put it, "We don't want to leave you girls with a bunch of clutter when we kick off.")

In the car, I turned on the radio and a Wham! song was playing—now a staple, I realized with a twinge, on the oldies station. As I drove, wearing my old jacket and singing along to George Michael, I passed the Burger King where I worked as a teen (the floor was so covered with grease and sesame seeds that we were instructed by the teen manager to skate rather than walk). Further down the road, I pass Hair We Are, the salon where I'd re-perm my perms when they got flat on top.

If, along with swimming, I take the Jazzercise classes that my Y still offers after many, many decades, my eighties time travel will be complete.

Other science-backed ways to lift your mood with movement, McGonigal writes, are moving outdoors, moving to music, moving through play or competition, such as sports and games, or moving with other people. My whole family loves a Manila-based YouTube fitness instructor named Keoni Tamayo, who does joyful low-impact workouts with his smiling mom as their rescue cats wander in and out of the room.

If you're experiencing brain fog after reading this chapter, I'll repeat for you, as a courtesy here, that this is likely to be temporary. "Data show that these mood changes ease with time after menopause," says Joffe. And if you treat your condition with antidepressants or other methods, she adds, you shouldn't expect to be on them for the rest of your life.

In the meantime, get help if you need it. If you are struggling, give yourself permission to seek support. I'm just going to keep saying it: the days of toughing it out in silence are over.

• Chapter 8 •

The Dry Vagina Monologues

It Shouldn't Hurt to Have Sex. Or Sit. Or Walk.

"This is why I can't help but get pissed," Dr. Maria Uloko is saying.

Uloko, an assistant professor of urology at UC San Diego School of Medicine, is also a urologist who specializes in female sexual dysfunction and menopause. She's been telling me about a patient of hers with symptoms of what was formerly known as vulvovaginal atrophy. In 2014, it was renamed as the less-depressing, zippier-sounding GSM, which sounds vaguely like a sports car but stands for genitourinary symptoms of menopause.

GSM, which afflicts a multitude of postmenopausal women—an estimated 50 to 70 percent—is a chronic condition that affects the vulva, vagina, and urinary tract. It also has a massive impact on your quality of life. Uloko's patient, a pianist and composer in her sixties, "hadn't been able to sit without pain and irritation until she came to us and we treated her," says Uloko. "That was her only goal—just to be able *sit comfortably*. Okay? And she had lived with this for twenty years."

As "reverse puberty" causes estrogen to leave your body, the skin that becomes markedly less supple, drier, and more sensitive includes tissues in your vagina, vulva, and urinary tract. Estrogen helps maintain the health of those tissues with blood flow, moisture, muscle function, and elasticity. So not only is sex painful as this area becomes more fragile, but very often, so are activities such as . . . wearing jeans. Or walking. Or wiping yourself with toilet paper. Or, you know, *sitting*.

"I'll walk into my office and a patient will be standing up, because their discomfort is such that they cannot sit down," says Dr. Makeba Williams of Washington University St. Louis. "I have patients that I've never seen wear pants."

The list of GSM symptoms is long: vaginal dryness, itching or burning, more discharge, and pelvic pain. Without estrogen, the walls of the urethra get weaker and thinner, too, lowering their defense against bacteria and increasing the risk of urinary tract infections. When the vagina and the bladder are dry, says Mary Jane Minkin of Yale Medical School, "there's nastier bacteria in the vagina, and bladder walls are more invadable, and that's why some women have their first UTI once they've gone through menopause. They may never have had one before."

These symptoms, per a 2020 overview of GSM in the medical journal *Cureus*, "rarely resolve spontaneously, and in most cases, deteriorate if left untreated." Yet many women have no idea that GSM *can* be treated. In a 2010 international survey entitled Women's Voices in the Menopause, over half of the U.S. participants didn't realize that local treatment was available for vaginal discomfort related to menopause. "To this day, GSM remains extremely underdiagnosed despite its high prevalence," asserts the *Cureus* review, "mostly because of the reluctance among women to seek help due to embarrassment, or as a result of a tendency among many women to consider it a normal feature of natural aging."

GSM's effect on the urinary tract often includes incontinence and having to pee more often. Women are much more prone in general to episodes of urine leakage than men, says NAMS's *Menopause Guidebook*, possibly because women have much shorter urethras—which shorten, in menopause, even further.

When I entered menopause, my urethra, which, admittedly, I've never measured, seemed to have shrunk to about a millimeter.

• • • •

A girl never forgets the first time she pees herself.

About two years ago, I became obsessed with being near a bathroom at all times. I'd worriedly scout for toilets every time I went out in public, just like I did when my daughter was a toddler. The minute I felt compelled to go, I had to race directly to a john or I'd pee my pants. I became familiar with every grimy bathroom in every gas station, drugstore, and grocery store within twenty miles of my town. More than once, I pulled over on a highway and dashed into the woods.

One warm spring day, I had just returned from—where else?—Stop & Shop, where I really should just set up a cot. If I'm not actually Stopping to Shop there, I have just Stopped or am preparing to Stop & Shop. I was doing a dance on the front steps of my house as I held a bag of groceries while simultaneously rooting through my purse, because I had to pee desperately. Where the hell were my keys?

I looked fearfully over my shoulder to see if any neighbors were watching. Where were the goddamn keys? Suddenly—*bloop!*—a river of urine gushed down my leg. When I finally got the door open, I took a shower, then hosed down my front steps, and told no one.

If, like me, you find yourself constantly sprinting to the bathroom, perhaps it's a small comfort that although we don't talk about it much, we are legion: research shows urinary incontinence affects over half of postmenopausal women.

GSM has a direct impact on your sex life, too. Thinner vaginal tissues can tear and bleed during sex, causing women to, understandably, avoid it. Penetration can feel like shards of glass are scraping your vagina, which is not exactly arousing. Vaginal secretions tend to diminish, too, so you are less lubricated.

Uloko specializes in treating what's known as genito-pelvic pain/penetration disorder, or the slightly clunky abbreviation GPPPD ("how many Ps are there, right?"). As she and her coauthor Dr. Rachel Rubin write in a 2021 study in the journal *Urologic Clinics of North America,* GPPPD is defined as at least six months of vulvovaginal or pelvic pain during penetrative sex, fear or anxiety around said pain in anticipation of penetration, and marked tensing or tightening of the pelvic floor muscles during penetration. This cycle of pain, they write, takes women by surprise, lowers their quality of life, and erodes their self-esteem. It also leads to "fear, hypervigilance in sexual situations or complete avoidance of sexual situations."

I know about the hypervigilance. Around the time of my rampant peeing jamboree, sex began to hurt—a lot. It felt like I was being exfoliated from the inside.

At the time, I had no clue that GPPPD even existed. Instead, I assumed that I had some sort of yeast infection—especially as that area was itchy and irritated, too—so I headed to the drugstore for some Monistat 3.

A week later, we tried again. Yee-*ouch*: the soreness was even

"People have the wrong assumption that [menopause] is when a woman stops being sexy. The concept of giving us an expiration date for everything based on your ability to create babies or not is really unfair. It should not define us as women. For so long, the concept of beauty in a woman was leaning completely to youth. And I think, 'Fuck that shit.'"

—Salma Hayek

worse. My cringing and grimacing were not exactly an aphrodisiac for Tom.

As our sex life withered, my magical thinking was that as the months went on, my soreness would somehow spontaneously resolve itself. It did not. I began to actively avoid Tom. I started creeping up to bed earlier than he did, and when I heard him trundling up the stairs—*crap, here he comes*—I'd quickly turn off the light, shove my book under the bed, and pretend I was asleep. I'd even do a little realistic heavy-but-not-too-heavy breathing.

Orgasms became a distant memory. This, too, is distressingly common. "I had a woman come to see me who told me that she lost her orgasm," says Rachel Rubin of Georgetown University Hospital. "She said, 'I used to taste color when I orgasmed, and I no longer have that feeling.' And I said, 'Well, if I could taste color when I orgasmed, and I lost that ability, I would also run to the doctor.'"

GPPPD was not a recognized disorder until 2013, when it appeared in the fifth edition of the *Diagnostic and Statistical Manual of Mental Disorders*, or DSM-5, used by clinicians. But most people still don't know what GPPPD is, let alone that it can be treated—and as Uloko and Rubin write, it's still a culturally taboo subject among many people that induces guilt and shame.

"GPPPD is excruciating, and really limits your quality of life," says Uloko. "Because now, every time you have sex, you associate it with pain, which drives a wedge into the whole narrative of being a sexually healthy person. Your partner is frustrated, you're frustrated."

The North American Menopause Society reports that up to 45 percent of postmenopausal women find sex painful. That's a pretty big number. But if a woman does bring up the issue of painful sex during a routine doctor's appointment, Uloko says, "what tends to happen is medical gaslighting. It's this incredibly common condition, yet women are being told, 'Nope, that's normal, it's *supposed* to be painful! Just have a glass of wine!' There's something wrong, but no one's acknowledging it, and instead, they're actually putting the blame on *you*."

Which is why Uloko is all fired up. "This needs to change," she says. "It's this really awful cycle that women go through, where there's lack of education on the provider side and then patients' lack of access to care and knowledge. There are just so many people who are in the dark about what can happen to their body. I make all my patients advocates. I tell them, 'The system has failed you. You should get angry. We should all be angry.'"

• • • •

Here's a compelling reason to get over any embarrassment around GSM and see a doctor: without treatment, vulvovaginal problems may not go away, says Yale's Mary Jane Minkin. "That's the really surprising thing that happens to many women—that the vaginal dryness may get worse over the course of time." At that point, they may not make the connection that it's GSM, Minkin adds. "Two or more years later after menopause, it's worse, and they say, 'Oh, shit, I did this menopause thing already, it must be something else.' And they imagine it can be all kinds of things."

As I chatted with these doctors, I realized that I could check the box for every single symptom of GSM. Fortunately, research shows GSM can be clinically detected by a doctor in up to 90 percent of postmenopausal women.

The first line of treatment for GSM—and the one I ultimately decided to use—is vaginal estrogen. The idea of hormones scares a lot of women—I'll get to that in the next chapter—but vaginal estrogen differs from oral hormone therapy in two important ways.

One is that it's applied topically, available in rings, creams, and inserts. For creams, you put a pea-sized dose into your vagina daily for the first two weeks, then a few times a week after that.

The other difference is that very low doses of estrogen are used. In fact, research shows that the amount of estrogen absorbed into the bloodstream with these vaginal forms is so small that the levels of estrogen in the blood are in the same range as that of postmenopausal women who *aren't* using vaginal estrogen.

A 2018 analysis of data from the Women's Health Initiative, which tracked about one hundred thousand women using vaginal estrogen creams or tablets, found that women who used vaginal estrogen had rates of endometrial cancer, invasive breast cancer, and deep vein thrombosis similar to those of nonusers (and in fact, the risks of coronary heart disease were lower in vaginal estrogen users). A 2020 study concluded that vaginal estrogen "may be considered safe in gynecologic cancer survivors." In a 2014 review of forty-four studies, vaginal estrogen was found to ably remedy all of GSM's major symptoms, including vaginal dryness, urinary incontinence, and painful penetration.

Low-dose vaginal estrogen has been shown to lower the risk of recurring UTIs, too, because estrogen restores the normal bacterial environment and acidic pH of the vagina, which limits the growth of unhealthy bacteria. Research published in 2021 in the journal *Female Pelvic Medicine & Reconstructive Surgery* found that vaginal estrogen worked so well for recurrent UTIs in postmenopausal women, 68 percent of them didn't need any other therapy.

But many women hear the word *estrogen* and won't even consider it. I was reticent myself until I read that many leading organizations and medical associations, among them NAMS and ACOG, which supports the use of vaginal estrogen for breast cancer survivors, have declared officially that vaginal estrogen is safe.

"As the research currently stands," announces the National Women's Health Network on its website, "it appears that vaginal estrogen is a safe and effective treatment for vaginal discomfort due to menopause, and has a much lower risk of the cancers and cardiovascular events typically associated with hormone therapy."

"No data shows a cancer with vaginal estrogen," echoes Rubin. "No. Data."

I am telling Dr. Rubin about peeing myself as I scramble to find the keys to my front door. "Oh my god, you're gonna get so much better if you take vaginal estrogen," she says. "It's crazy." I say that I had no idea vaginal estrogen could help with incontinence. "Oh, yeah. You'll see. Just know that local hormones take at least two to three months to work. You don't water a plant that's already dead and expect it to grow. Right?"

I am convinced.

I had a thorough exam with my ob-gyn, who prescribed me vaginal estradiol, which has been around for decades. (Like my teenage daughter, my ob-gyn would prefer not to be mentioned, which I will respect.)

When I brought the tube home from the pharmacy, I was alarmed by the all-caps warning emblazoned on the box, alerting users of the risk of ENDOMETRIAL CANCER, CARDIOVASCULAR DISORDERS, BREAST CANCER, AND PROBABLE DEMENTIA. Probable dementia?

This "black box" warning is applied by the FDA to any estrogen-containing pharmaceutical, "and understandably frightens patients," says Nanette Santoro of the University of Colorado School of Medicine. She is one of many prominent women's health experts who say that these risks have not been substantiated. Dr. Santoro and a long list of fellow physicians, along with various organizations such as NAMS, have been lobbying the FDA to get rid of what Santoro calls "that scary, awful labeling" on topical estrogen formulas, but the FDA has so far refused.

After three months of assiduously applying my vaginal estrogen, I had the equivalent of a new-model vag. Sex had almost entirely stopped hurting (bolstered by liberal lashings of lube). Going to the bathroom was no longer a desperate sprint. My nighttime episodes of waking up to pee were reduced to once a night, down from three or four. Toilet paper no longer felt like medium-grit sandpaper. The only side effect I had was breast tenderness, a symptom I experienced in perimenopause that faded once I hit menopause. It returned for about three months, but my ob-gyn told me it would abate. It did.

The remaining downside is that I must take it indefinitely. If I stop, the symptoms come back. Another thing to keep in mind when using vaginal estrogen therapy, says Lauren Streicher of Northwestern University, is that while it can help your vaginal tissues, the underlying muscles may still rebel. "Some women report that they still have painful sex even after diligently applying vaginal estrogen, and will give up," says Streicher. "They'll think it isn't working, so they abandon it—but it *is* working on the tissue. But often what happens during sex is that your pelvic muscles, including the muscles surrounding the opening of the vagina, will involuntarily contract. The medical word for this is *vaginismus*. Your vagina's not stupid—and if sex hurts like hell, your vagina is going to tell your brain, 'Don't go there.'"

If this is you, Streicher says that in addition to treating the tissue with a local vaginal estrogen, treat the underlying muscles by using vaginal dilators (see below) or pelvic floor physical therapy. (While she's on the subject, Streicher says that if you need help having an orgasm, try applying vaginal estrogen cream directly to the clitoris, which she says can potentially aid orgasms by directing blood flow to the area.)

GSM can also be addressed with systemic hormones like patches or pills, says Minkin, but about 20 percent of people who do so will still need a vaginal estrogen booster.

For those who aren't candidates for vaginal estrogen, or don't want to take it, there are other options.

The one FDA-approved oral medication for GSM is called **ospemifene** (known by the brand name Osphena). Ospemifene is a SERM, or selective estrogen receptor modulator, a class of drugs that bind to estrogen receptors in your body and can mimic the effect of estrogen. A daily oral tablet originally formulated to stop bone thinning, ospemifene has been shown to help fortify vaginal tissue in three months.

DHEA (dehydroepiandrosterone), meanwhile, is a hormone that is transformed intracellularly to estrogen in the bloodstream. It's FDA-approved to treat sexual pain and vaginal dryness in those with GSM. Also known as prasterone, it's a vaginal insert that needs to be administered daily.

Laser therapy, which uses laser and energy-based devices to regenerate vaginal tissues, is very promising, but it's not yet FDA-approved for GSM and more studies are needed.

The Menopause Guidebook from NAMS states that when basic measures fail, **Botox** can also "be injected into the bladder walls to reduce urgency."

As for options that are cheap and free, good old **masturbation** stimulates blood flow and natural moisture, which makes your vaginal tissues more elastic. ACOG recommends masturbation as a remedy for painful sex. Self-love is self-care!

Out of practice? Guided masturbation apps such as Ferly,

founded by two women, has detailed audio guides for self-touch. They specifically made this science-based app for people who struggle with sex issues, whether it's feeling disconnected and unable to get in the mood, finding that sex is painful mentally or physically, or having difficulties with orgasm.

Dr. Barb DePree, a gynecologist and renowned menopause specialist in Holland, Michigan, often recommends vibrators to her menopausal patients. "One of the best treatments for prevention of progressive loss of vulvovaginal integrity is having sex, whether it's partnered or solo," she says. For maximum health benefit, the vibrator should be inserted vaginally, adds DePree. "The action of penetrative sex brings blood supply to the genitals, improves lubrication, and keeps muscles more toned."

And orgasms, DePree says, are good for women's health in midlife. "Orgasm is contraction of the pelvic floor muscles, and this action is very beneficial for the ongoing strength and health of the pelvic floor," she says. "It has been shown this also improves immunity, reduces chronic pain, and improves sleep and mood."

To replenish moisture, try **vaginal moisturizers** and **vaginal lubricants**. There are key differences between the two, says New York City ob-gyn Kameelah Phillips. Vaginal moisturizers, she says, are designed to replace natural vaginal secretions and meant to be used daily "to help bring and trap moisture in the area, and to make the tissue a little bit more plump and less sensitive to daily irritation."

Vaginal moisturizers commonly contain molecules capable of retaining large amounts of water. Dr. Minkin recommends Replens, an over-the-counter gel; Dr. Phillips recommends a vaginal suppository called Revaree, which contains hyaluronic acid, a substance found naturally throughout the body. As mentioned in chapter 6, each molecule of HA can attract and retain up to a thousand times its weight in moisture, so it can nicely hydrate fragile vaginal tissue.

(An aside here: You may not see ads for these lubricants on Facebook, because Facebook classifies them as "adult" products—although somehow, ads for male libido-enhancing products have squeaked through.)

A more natural moisturizing option, says Phillips, are oils such as coconut oil or olive oil. "If you find that you don't have any irritation to the oils," she says, "people commonly use them, and they work."

Vaginal lubricants, meanwhile, are typically water-based but contain additional silicone, oil, or glycerin. "Lubricants are used to decrease friction," says Phillips, "which happens especially during intercourse, or things like jogging, when you really need a slip on the vagina to make more intense activity more comfortable."

The most delicate tissue in the body is the vulvovaginal tissue, Dr. Minkin puts in, so lay off any fragranced products, "and if you're buying lubricant for the first time, don't buy the economy size, because your body may be sensitive to it and then you've wasted your money."

Phillips sometimes suggests that menopausal patients take a **probiotic with lactobacillus.** A 2016 study of the menopausal vaginal microbiome in the medical journal *Maturitas* says that while probiotics need more research, they show "great promise" in alleviating menopausal symptoms such as vaginal dryness. **Vaginal dilators, or vaginal trainers,** are tube-shaped devices in various sizes (and sometimes festive colors). They're made of plastic or soft silicone and are used to gently and gradually expand the vagina. Streicher says they are a therapeutic tool with two purposes: to get the vagina used to having something inside it, and to erase the muscle memory that has kept your pelvic floor in protective mode during painful

"Many people think after menopause, women give up the idea of sex. For me, sex since then has been better because you don't need to worry about pregnancy. Right now I have a boyfriend who is twenty-one years younger. I see sex as a necessary balance along with good food, humor, joy for life."

—artist Marina Abramović

sex. By starting small and then slowly increasing the size of the dilators, she says, the vaginal tissues and pelvic floor muscles "learn" to accommodate having something inside without triggering a pain response.

"Every time you stretch the vagina with vaginal dilators, blood flow improves, elasticity improves, moisture improves," adds Dr. Lubna Pal of Yale Medicine. "I mean, we put so much attention to our face and our hands. What about the vagina?"

For incontinence, **Kegel exercises**, or contracting and relaxing the pelvic floor muscles, can help. You can find your pelvic floor muscles by tensing the muscles that would normally stop the flow of pee while you're sitting on the toilet—those are the ones you'll strengthen during Kegel exercises. You can also put your finger into your vagina and squeeze the muscles around it—the ones you feel "lifting" inside of you are your pelvic floor muscles. ("Think of your pelvic floor as an elevator, and raise that elevator up," instructs Dr. Minkin.)

Start by lifting and holding your pelvic floor muscles for three seconds, then relaxing. Repeat the contract/relax cycle ten times. Try to do thirty to forty Kegel exercises a day. You can do them in public—in line at the bank, in your car while you're stopped at a red light—and no one will know.

While we're on the subject of urine flow, Minkin supplies another useful exercise for the many women who "say they pee, think they're empty, then get up and two minutes later they feel like they have to go again, which is very common," she says. (This is my life.) Practice what urologists call a **double void technique**. "Pee, sit there for a couple of minutes and look at your cell phone or whatever, pee again, and then leave," says Minkin. "Build that into your routine."

For stray leakage, you may be tempted to use maxi-pads rather than incontinence pads. "We found a lot of people were doing that when we started digging into the data," says Beatrice Dixon, founder of The Honey Pot Company. But according to the nonprofit organization the National Association for Continence (their entirely winning campaign slogan: *Life's More Fun Without Leaks!*), incontinence pads are designed to absorb and hold much more fluid than menstrual pads, and they have better skin protection against acidic urine.

"Look, incontinence happens to everybody," states Dixon in the forthright way that I want to emulate. "And we want to support people in their vaginal journey—or, okay, their urinary journey."

• • • •

If you have a partner with whom you're intimate, have a clear, candid discussion about what is going on with your body. It may be uncomfortable, but here is what is more uncomfortable: pretending that sex doesn't feel like shards of glass are methodically scraping away at your vaginal lining!

"You have had a biological change, and your body is not the same body as it was before menopause," says Georgetown's Rubin. "This is biology. This is physiology."

If you are shying away from sex, avoiding it outright, or glumly enduring it, your partner has likely sensed your reticence; without an explanation, they may be hurt, angry, or assume that your relationship is in trouble.

Talk to your partner and tell them what is going on with your body—and how, specifically, they can help you though this. Give them a way forward and a plan, which will help you both. "When I teach the biology to patients, their partners say, 'Oh, thank god, I thought I was crazy, or that she wasn't attracted to me anymore,'" says Rubin. "Communication is so important, because the idea that somehow you're supposed to inherently come preprogrammed to know how your partner's buttons work is insanity."

It's just as important—no, it is imperative—that you talk to a doctor if you have GSM. While vaginal irritation and leaky bladders may be "normal" in menopause, that doesn't mean it's optimal. Why should you live with not being able to wear pants—unless they're the MC Hammer style dropped-crotch ones where the fabric is at least a foot away from your inflamed vulva? Why should you have to look around to make sure no one is watching at the gym so you can do a furtive labial scratch, because your workout clothes are making your vulva unbearably itchy? Why should you have to dread hugging your partner because it might lead to sex, an activity that once brought you pleasure? Why should you resignedly toss yet another pee-soaked pair of underwear into the clothes hamper?

"If another part of your body hurt, you would take care of it," says Phillips. "If you had a toothache, you wouldn't *not* take care of the toothache. You would address it. And we have to remove the taboo around the vagina aching. It's a body part! It has function—and when it starts to lose function and causes discomfort, getting it treated should be normalized."

Make no mistake: These are medical problems that deeply affect your quality of life. Dr. Rubin says she is constantly amazed at how differently we approach women's sexual health compared to men. "As a urologist, I'm taught to give a shit about quality of life," she says. "When a man comes to the doctor for a change in sexual function or how he's urinating or anything affecting his quality of life, no one blinks an eye."

Not so with women, she goes on. "We *never* lead with quality of life. We are always talking about risk reducing—will this kill you, will you get cancer, will this hurt the baby? We do not talk about quality of life in women. We don't even have the vocabulary to do that. It's just crazy how much work we have to do."

So give yourself permission, say Uloko and Rubin, to see a specialist. "The idea that your ob-gyn is the only one responsible for this is nothing short of systemic misogyny," says Rubin. "We collectively just want to push off all of women's healthcare on this one field of medicine, but the idea that ob-gyns should be menopause experts and specialists, along with delivering babies, cancer surgery, doing pap smears and mammograms and everything else, is actually kind of terrible, and also not feasible. There's no doctor for men that is supposed to do everything! It doesn't exist!"

Yes, a specialist costs money that may or may not be reimbursed by insurance, but Rubin says that given all the time and copays women squander on fruitless doctor visits, as well as "all the shitty advice they've gotten," a specialist can be worth the money.

"It's not like I provide magic in terms of a new prescription or therapy that patients don't know about or can't read about," Rubin says. "What I do provide is lots of time and education and treatment that's tailored to a patient's specific story. Like, that's the magic. And that's the thing that is so hard to find."

When patients visit Uloko, they are often worn out and desperate. She takes a thorough medical history as well as a detailed exam and labs. "I have a very high cure rate," Uloko says. "It's a lot of exploration, education, and advocacy, and letting patients know, 'What has happened to you is not normal, and we're going to fix this. It's not going to happen overnight, and it's going to take a team approach, but we're going to fix this.'"

When patients come back to Rubin a few months later, she says, they tell her: *Holy shit, it's about wearing pants again*. "Bare minimum, you should be able to wear pants," she says. "This is about normal acts of daily living."

Low libido may be not a physical problem, but a psychological one—or a combination of both. If sex, either with a partner or with yourself, once gave you pleasure but has significantly degraded during menopause, pay attention, advises Dr. Hope Ashby, a Los Angeles psychologist, sex therapist, and life coach.

"In many cases, women inherently know that there's something amiss," says Ashby. She lists some warning signs. "Maybe you used to masturbate, and now you don't, or you used to have sex regularly with your partner, and now you don't," she says. "When it comes to the quality of your orgasms, it may not be fireworks anymore—it may just be sort of like a poof, or you're not having them at all. Or maybe when you used to watch a show and see Idris Elba, Chris Hemsworth, or J.Lo, you'd get a little of what I call the 'clitoral twitch'—and you're not getting it anymore."

If you're mourning the loss of your sexuality, and saddened that Idris Elba prompts a clitoral flatline, you deserve to have a healthy sex life.

"Recognize that shift and confront it head-on," instructs Dr. Ashby. Find a provider, she suggests, that is not just a gynecologist but a specialist in women's sexual health. They can help you address medical, social, psychological, and cultural issues that are causing your low libido.

An expert, she continues, can ask questions that an ob-gyn may not, such as: Has the quality of your orgasms changed? Are you enjoying sex anymore? Are you lubricating enough? Are you feeling anxiety around the idea of sex? Have you checked your testosterone levels? Are you with a partner who is open to helping you get there when it comes to orgasms, if it takes longer than it used to?

"This is a time in your life when you can truly be a free sexual being," points out Ashby. "You don't have to worry about pregnancy, or periods, or the ridiculous price of tampons and pads."

• • • •

When I first started using vaginal estrogen, I followed Rubin's advice and talked to Tom during one of our afternoon walks. I explained that as estrogen was leaving my body, my physiology was changing.

"You've probably noticed that I tense up when you give me hugs," I told him. "That's not because I don't care about you. Lately, I'm just afraid of a hug leading to something more . . ."

"Carnal?" he supplied.

"Right. And my vaginal tissues are fragile without the estrogen and I've even bled a little bit after sex."

He nodded. "So that's why you've been faking sleep when I stay up later than you?"

"You knew?"

He laughed. "Of course I knew! You're a terrible actor. I just figured you didn't want to have sex anymore. I mean, over the years, your sex life goes up and down, so to speak."

"But you assumed this was going down for good?"

He shook his head. "I didn't know. It's not like you ever go through the same stage of life twice, so you have no idea of what's normal or not normal unless you ask people. Which is the last thing I'd ever talk about with someone."

I recalled what Dr. Rubin said about giving him a way forward. I told him I was trying vaginal estrogen, stocking up on lubes and moisturizers, and would try to be transparent with him. "I'd love if you could be patient with me, because apparently the estrogen takes two or three months to work. And let me know if you feel upset or rejected. We can do other things aside from penetrative sex." I borrow Dr. Rubin's phrase. "It's not you. It's just biology. It's just physiology."

As we walked on, I asked him how he knew I was faking sleep.

"Because in real life, you snore," he said.

· Chapter 9 ·

Hormone Therapy—Let's Go There

Life-Restoring Miracle? Rife with Risks? Both? Neither?

I'm in my ob-gyn's office near my home in New Jersey, awaiting an exam. I have on a blue gown and nothing else.

Some people get what is known as white-coat syndrome in a physician's office, in which their blood pressure spikes when they're around doctors, who often sport white coats. I always have low-level jitters during doctor visits, but I also find their offices soothing: the deep quiet, broken only by murmuring voices outside the door; the earnest posters (*Understanding the Female Reproductive System*); the faint smell of rubbing alcohol.

Not everyone, to say the least, is lulled, as I am, by this atmosphere. In 2021, an Indiana urogynecologist named Ryan Stewart announced on Twitter that he was designing his office at the Midwest Center for Pelvic Health from scratch, and asked people what they would change to "optimize a visit to the gynecologist's office."

Stewart finished his post with "If I've ever had a tweet worthy of virality, it's this one."

He was correct. Thousands of suggestions flooded in. *"Please please no TV in the waiting room, it's stressful and noisy." "Please have images of Black women in the office. I haven't visited a gynecologist office yet with this type of representation." "Appropriately sized cloth gowns, no tiny paper sheet shirts." "Please consider not asking the patient if an intern can be in the room in the presence of the intern. It's hard to say no in front of them." "Don't discuss care or diagnoses while people are naked." "A wide variety of speculum sizes." "The crotch end of the bed NOT directed at the door."*

One person pointed out that not only were stirrup warmers a bonus, but they presented an opportunity for comedy. (Her doctor had warmers over the stirrups that said I HATE on one and THIS PART on the other, another was emblazoned with ARE WE and DONE YET?.)

I agree with every one of those comments. I find waiting-room TVs stressful, too: blaring news reports of the latest horrible crime jangle your nerves as you're tensely waiting for mammogram results. And I've been in many exam rooms where my legs face an open door so that I'm showing my business to anyone who strolls by. I'd also suggest losing the headache-inducing fluorescent lights.

When my feet are in the stirrups, I must always stifle the urge to say, *Go on now, giddyap*, or look around gravely and announce: *Gentlemen, get thee to bed, for tomorrow we leave at first light.* Once a high school class clown, always a class clown ("Wackiest Wit," Chatham Township High School class of '84).

I am at my ob-gyn's office to discuss if menopausal hormone therapy, or MHT, is right for me. (It's no longer called hormone replacement therapy, NAMS medical director Stephanie Faubion told *The Washington Post*, because the purpose is not to *replace* what the ovary once made or to use the hormones indefinitely, but to manage menopause symptoms.)

MHT is used to treat common symptoms, such as hot flashes and vaginal dryness, with estrogen—and, for women with a uterus, the addition of progestin, a synthetic hormone that mimics progesterone. (Estrogen alone can stimulate growth of the lining of the uterus, increasing the risk of endometrial cancer, while estrogen with progestin does not.)

The pros and cons of MHT are a complicated and divisive issue—particularly after a bomb dropped on the world of women's health in July of 2002. It was then that the Women's Health Initiative, an unusually large long-term national health study that focused on strategies for preventing heart disease, breast cancer, and osteoporosis in women who were postmenopausal, released some distressing news.

The two randomized clinical trials, sponsored by the National Institutes of Health, had enrolled more than 27,000 healthy women aged fifty to seventy-nine. The goal of the trials was to see if MHT prevented bone fracture and heart disease. One group, women with a uterus, was randomly assigned estrogen plus progestin or a placebo; the other group of women, who did not have a uterus, was assigned estrogen alone or a placebo.

Researchers found that the women in the study who were taking hormones had a higher risk of breast cancer (26 percent) as well as a higher risk of heart disease, stroke, and deep vein thrombosis than the women in the study who received placebos. Given those risks, the WHI announced, the study would be halted prematurely.

Panic ensued. Reaction was swift. "I really would not have wanted to be in a fish in the United States on July 10, 2002, the day after the WHI's announcement," says Mary Jane Minkin of Yale Medical School. "Because I'm convinced that all women went to their toilets and promptly flushed down any estrogenic substances they had in their house."

Not all the news was bad. All the women in the original study who took hormones were found to have a reduced risk of diabetes, colorectal cancer, fractures, and what is known as all-cause mortality, or death from any cause.

It didn't matter. Within months, use of hormone therapy plummeted by half.

• • • •

A half-century ago, the use of menopausal hormone therapy was widespread. One of the pioneering drugs for MHT was, as mentioned earlier, Premarin, introduced in 1941 and made from a mix of estrogen compounds extracted from pregnant mare urine, which company researchers found was similar to human estrogens. It's still made that way today, and animal activist groups such as People for the Ethical Treatment of Animals (PETA) contend that pregnant mares are kept confined for long periods of time in narrow stalls to collect their urine. Some avoid Premarin for that reason alone.

MHT received a robust boost by physician Robert A. Wilson, who penned a 1966 bestseller, *Feminine Forever*, in which he deemed menopause a "disease." Wilson was commendably adept at scare language. One of "the saddest of human spectacles," he wrote, describing the Change, was the "horror of this living decay." Without hormone therapy, Wilson insinuated, women would look like King Tut's mummy when the sarcophagus was pried open. Later it was revealed that Wilson had apparently accepted funds from the pharmaceutical company that made the hormones he was espousing.

By 1975, Premarin was the fifth-most-prescribed drug in the United States. Soon after, MHT's reputation took a hit when

"Having that hormone support allows me to have that energy to do anything, okay? I want to climb the mountain."

–Trinny Woodall

reports of a four to fourteen times increased risk of endometrial cancers was linked to estrogen therapy, and the FDA slapped a warning on all estrogen products indicating a risk for cancer and blood clots. In the 1980s, researchers discovered that lowering the dose of estrogen and combining it with progesterone reduced the risk of endometrial cancer, and the use of MHT surged once again.

Then came the WHI's 2002 announcement.

Since then, the WHI's results have been endlessly analyzed. Detractors point out the many limitations of the study. The average age of participants in the WHI who started hormone therapy was sixty-three—a full dozen years after the average age of menopause.

Subjects weren't necessarily in the peak of health, either. "A fifth were between the ages of seventy and seventy-nine," says Minkin. "And half were current or former smokers." A reanalysis of the WHI trial with women aged fifty to fifty-nine, for instance, found that those on MHT had a reduction in myocardial infarction, or heart attacks.

JoAnn Manson, chief of preventative medicine at Brigham & Women's Hospital and a lead investigator in the WHI, has pointed out that the WHI was examining hormone therapy *not* as a way to manage menopause symptoms like hot flashes, but to see whether MHT could be taken long term to stave off certain chronic diseases. While the research "does not support the use of HT for prevention of chronic disease purposes," Manson wrote in the journal *Women's Health*, "I believe that one message is that the short-term use of HT to manage moderate-to-severe hot flashes or other symptoms in early menopause remains appropriate—the WHI has provided evidence for that."

In both trials (estrogen alone and estrogen with progesterone), Manson maintained, "the quality-of-life outcomes with HT were mixed, with reduced vasomotor symptoms (e.g., hot flashes), improved sleep and joint pain, but increased breast tenderness. However, the benefits are likely to outweigh the risks for many women seeking treatment for their symptoms during the menopause transition." Moreover, "the WHI demonstrates that the absolute risk of adverse events is much lower in younger than older women."

Further studies directly examining MHT as a way to manage menopause symptoms are reinforcing the view that it's highly beneficial when given to healthy women within ten years of menopause or those who are under sixty (known as the critical window hypothesis).

As the authors write in a 2018 review of the research in *American Journal of Physiology: Heart and Circulatory Physiology*, "it is increasingly apparent that postmenopausal MHT has cardiovascular and cognitive benefits, provided it is initiated within the critical window of opportunity, i.e. [within ten years of menopause] and it has even better outcomes if 1) it is initiated perimenopausally, 2) it is administered transdermally." (As in not a pill, but instead, for example, a patch.)

NAMS's position statement on MHT, endorsed by health organizations around the world, from the American Society for Reproductive Medicine to the South African Menopause Society, is that it "remains the most effective treatment for vasomotor and genitourinary symptoms of menopause, and has been shown to prevent bone loss and fracture." (And who knew that hormone therapy may even extend to reducing gum disease, per a University of Buffalo study?)

Question marks undoubtedly remain, and so do risks. For women under sixty, the NAMS statement goes on, those risks include higher rates of breast cancer with combined estrogen-progesterone therapy, endometrial cancer if estrogen is unopposed, deep vein thrombosis, stroke, heart attacks, and dementia. This does sound scary. But "absolute attributable risk for women in the 50 to 59-year age group is low," asserts NAMS's position statement.

And the benefits, NAMS's statement goes on to say, include "relief of bothersome vasomotor symptoms, prevention of bone loss for women at high risk for fracture, treatment of genitourinary syndrome, and improved sleep, well-being, and quality of life." Further, breast cancer risk, per NAMS, usually doesn't rise until after about five years with estrogen-progesterone therapy or after seven years with estrogen alone.

Leading ob-gyn and certified menopause practitioner Sharon Malone put the risk in perspective in a 2022 op-ed in *The Washington Post*: "Further research has shown the link [of MHT] to breast cancer to be minimal—statistically less than the risk incurred by working as a flight attendant or by drinking two glasses of wine at dinner nightly."

The pendulum seems to have swung from the idea that hormone therapy should be mandatory to "hormone therapy is poison" to a place somewhere in between. "There are real risks of hormone therapy, for sure," says Camille Moreno of Duke University Medical Center. "But we have a better understanding that for the right woman, at the right time, and for the right indications, hormone therapy is safe and effective."

It's worth noting that, according to Northwestern University's Lauren Streicher, "virtually every female academic menopause expert I know, including me, takes hormone therapy."

Mary Jane Minkin of Yale Medical School is seeing "a real turning point" in which more of her younger patients are open to MHT. "We have a whole lot of young women in their forties who are getting perimenopausal symptoms and beginning to feel like crap," she says. "And they didn't hear about the Women's Health

Initiative. They're not sleeping, they're getting hot, their skin's getting dry, they don't like it. And they're saying, 'What do you mean, you can't do anything for me?' They want relief and they want it now."

Of course, the choice to take MHT is a highly personal one. Among the factors to help you in your decision, according to the Cleveland Clinic, are your age, family history, personal medical history, and the severity of your menopausal symptoms. Are your hot flashes a nuisance, or are they so bad that you haven't slept in months and you feel deranged?

• • • •

If you're considering MHT, have your doctor do a full medical exam and screening, including a blood pressure check, a test for diabetes, and screenings for cholesterol and breast cancer.

Your medical history should be just as thorough. That includes your personal and family history of heart disease, stroke, cancer, gynecologic cancer, blood clots, liver disease, and osteoporosis.

Before you meet with your doctor, research how many of your relatives, including so-called second-degree relatives such as grandparents, cousins, and great-aunts, have been diagnosed with breast cancer. If you're able, find out how old they were when diagnosed and what sort of treatment they had. (As I mentioned earlier, "balance" app can also help you figure out your risk profile.) Then you can carefully go over the pros and cons with your doctor.

MHT is known as systemic therapy, meaning that it sends hormones into your bloodstream so they can travel throughout your whole body. The amount and potency of hormones in MHT is dramatically lower than in birth control pills. MHT can be given in pills or transdermally, meaning on the skin. ACOG's website maintains that transdermal therapy, via a patch, gel, vaginal ring, or spray, is associated with less risk of complications from stroke, blood clots, and gallbladder disease than oral forms of MHT.

A quick note here: If you're using a spray, which is usually applied to your forearm, best not to do it in front of a fireplace. Or a kid. Sprays such as Evamist are alcohol-based, so they can be flammable. "Avoid fire, flame or smoking until the spray has dried," states the warning. Young children who are accidentally exposed as you mist away, it goes on, "may show signs of puberty that are not expected."

If you haven't had your uterus removed, your doctor will typically prescribe estrogen along with progesterone or progestin, which is a synthetic medication that mimics progesterone. If you've had your uterus removed, you may not need to take progestin.

MHT can be pricey if your health insurance plan is like mine and doesn't pay for prescription drugs. Often you can find options within your insurance company that they will cover, says Rachel Rubin of Georgetown. She passes on a few cost-saving tips. Create an account with the company Costplusdrugs.com, she instructs. Have your doctor send a prescription to the website's electronic medical record, and the company can order generic versions of hormone preparations such as vaginal estrogen inserts, creams, or patches for much lower prices. "Super inexpensive, super incredible," Rubin adds. Another possibility, as mentioned, is to check out the website goodrx.com and look for cost-saving coupons at your local pharmacy.

If you're perimenopausal, taking—or continuing to take—an oral contraceptive pill can manage symptoms like hot flashes, night sweats, and chaotic periods. (I have always assumed that this is the most popular form of birth control, but according to government data from 2020, the Pill is used by only 14 percent of sexually active women age fifteen to forty-nine. The most popular form of birth control is actually sterilization, or having your tubes tied.)

If you reach menopause and are still experiencing symptoms, you can transition from the Pill into MHT, which, again, uses smaller doses of hormones. (Higher amounts are needed to suppress ovulation.) If you are on the Pill, know that it may not be entirely clear to you when you've officially reached menopause.

As treatment should be individualized, the process to find the right medication and dosage for MHT may involve trial and error—sometimes a lot of trial and error. And every year, per ACOG, people should check in with their doctor to assess whether to continue treatment.

"If you're in good health and if you are having severe menopause symptoms that are affecting your quality of life, don't just grin and bear it," says Wen Shen of Johns Hopkins. "Because we do have evidence to show that women who have severe menopause symptoms may have abnormalities in their cardiovascular system and that their blood pressures go up during a hot flash. So these women may be at increased risk for cardiovascular disease." Shen thinks for a moment. "Or if, say, in your family history, your mom had her first heart attack when she was sixty or broke her hip when she was sixty, then it would behoove you to consider MHT."

Here's one point that Holland, Michigan, gynecologist and menopause practitioner Barb DePree makes to patients that usually gets them to think a bit differently about hormones: "For forty years, we all have an abundance of estrogen and progesterone circulating in our systems on an ongoing basis, and no one ever suggests we are in harm's way because of this.

"So why, when you turn fifty-two, does this thing that has been great for you now suddenly cause risk or harm?" she goes on. "I reject that notion. I also mention to women that to my knowledge, it is the only human condition that has expected organ failure—as in, menopause's ovarian failure—and we choose to ignore it. Then we discuss the timing of initiation and underlying risk factors."

Evidence suggests that there are important differences in breast cancer risk depending on the form of progesterone you use. The WHI study used medroxyprogesterone acetate, a synthetic progesterone, but a 2022 study in the journal *Obstetrics & Gynecology* found that taking micronized bioidentical progesterone with estrogen was safer.

An optimal combination, according to a 2019 editorial in the *British Journal of General Practice*, is micronized bioidentical progesterone and transdermal estrogen, which is not associated with an increased risk of venous thromboembolism (blood clots). As the authors wrote, "there is no increased risk of breast cancer for the first five years of taking estrogen with micronized progesterone." While you're weighing pros and cons, one consideration is this: If you're suffering persistent lack of sleep thanks to hot flashes and night sweats, this alone can have serious health consequences, both mental and physical. Chronic sleep loss over time can lead to cardiovascular disease, type 2 diabetes, and depression. For those who feel their mental and physical health declining from ongoing sleep loss, MHT can be life-changing. A friend of mine said that after her hormone therapy had kicked in, she woke up one morning and wept with relief when she realized that she had slept through the night for the first time in three years.

My ob-gyn was commendably thorough during our appointment to discuss MHT: I was in her office for over an hour. Per my experts' advice, I booked a separate appointment to discuss MHT, rather than shoehorn it into a wellness visit. If you're considering hormone therapy, it's vital to take the lead, rather than waiting for your doctor to bring it up.

As my ob-gyn and I delved into my medical history and she asked if I've ever had various diseases, I felt grateful every time I answered no. I told her that the main reason I wanted to go on MHT was to regulate my sleep. I kept thinking about my friend's tears upon waking: sleeping though the night seemed unimaginable.

But near the end of our meeting, when we shifted into family history, I told her that one of my sisters has been hospitalized twice for what are known as "unprovoked" blood clots. ("Provoked" is where there is an identifiable trigger for the clot, like an injury, whereas an unprovoked one happens seemingly out of the blue.) When I disclosed this, she looked up sharply. I showed her my sister's hospital records. (At that point, it had been drilled in my head by experts to be hyper-prepared.)

She told me that while going on MHT was ultimately my choice, because my sister was a first-degree relative experiencing blood clots, along with my family history of strokes, she advised against it. I would have preferred to take care of most of my worst symptoms in one go with MHT; instead, I'd have to continue to tackle them in piecemeal fashion.

And I had already made progress. As I said in the previous chapter, the effects of my vaginal estrogen had fully kicked in. I don't throw around the term *life-changing* lightly, but it's a straight-up miracle to me that a cream that you apply to your vagina can *make you stop peeing yourself.* When I'm in any sort of public place, my first thought is no longer *Welp, might as well pee while I'm here.* My sleep, in fact, has already improved, because I don't get up to visit the john multiple times a night. I will happily apply vaginal estrogen forever.

Sex, as mentioned, is no longer a nightmare, either. I'd estimate that my sexual pain, thanks to vaginal estrogen, is 90 percent gone—and I've been able to take care of the remaining soreness with lube. I've been using vaginal suppositories called "intimacy melts," which are infused with 50 milligrams of CBD and made by a company called Foria. Stick them in 15 minutes before sex, and they melt to "ease discomfort and increase relaxation." (You can use them to soothe discomfort post-sex, too.)

I know the research on CBD is still emerging, but these "melts" work for me—and this is my message throughout this book. If something works for you, that is all that matters. As a science reporter, I favor clinical studies and hard data, but in some cases, a menopausal remedy hasn't been well studied. That doesn't mean it's not effective.

When it comes to my "melts" and other treatments, it could be that the placebo effect—when your brain convinces your body that a fake treatment has real results—is making me feel better. In recent years, science has found that the mind-body connection is so strong that given the right circumstances, a placebo can deliver the same effect as a traditional treatment—particularly for conditions like pain management.

Usually, in randomized controlled trials, participants don't know if they're getting a placebo or a medication. But in a study published in 2014 in the journal *Science Translational Medicine*, researchers tested to see how people reacted to migraine pain medication when they had a migraine attack. One group took a migraine drug labeled with the drug's name, Maxalt. Another group took nothing. The third group took a placebo pill that was actually labeled "placebo"—it's called an open label placebo. The results? The advertised placebo was 50 percent as effective as the real drug to dial down pain after a migraine attack—and anyone who has ever weathered a migraine knows that its throbbing agony is no joke.

The researchers speculated that one reason might be that the simple act of taking a pill—even a clearly labeled fake one—had a positive healing effect. "Even if they know it's not medicine," said Ted Kaptchuk, one of the investigators, "the action itself can stimulate the brain into thinking the body is being healed."

* * * *

While I'm on the subject of hard data, a word here about compounded bioidentical hormones. In recent years, so-called bioidentical hormones have ballooned in popularity as a more natural alternative to conventional MHT.

Bioidentical refers to compounds that claim to be chemically and molecularly identical to the ones your body produces. The idea, says ob-gyn Barb DePree, is that "with bioidenticals, you end up with a molecule that is exactly like human hormones, whereas non-bioidentical hormones are similar but not identical."

Instead of being manufactured by a multinational pharmaceutical company, they're typically prescribed by a clinician and then custom-compounded by a pharmacy that specializes in making meds that are tailored to individuals—so they are touted as safer. The internet is buzzing with testimonies from celebrities and influencers extolling the benefits of bioidentical hormones (some with claims of eternal youth, such as shiny hair, radiant skin, and better muscle tone). And business is booming—fueled, among other things, by the public's distrust for Big Pharma and the belief that natural is better.

Bioidentical hormone replacement therapy, says DePree, "is not a miracle cure, a fountain of youth, or some kind of snake oil concocted by unscrupulous doctors. The truth is much more nuanced." Menopausal hormone therapy, she says, "is intended neither to keep your hormones 'in harmony' nor to keep menopause at bay

"[Menopause] is as natural as having a child. It really is: it's part of life. Physically, it's part of how we're made; hormonally, it's how we're constructed; chemically, it's how we work."

—Kim Cattrall

indefinitely. Hormone therapy is intended to ease the symptoms of the menopause transition when they are interfering with your life."

While custom-compounded hormones are undoubtedly popular—a 2015 NAMS survey revealed that one in three current users of MHT is using compounded hormone therapy—they are decidedly not safer.

In fact, compounded drugs are neither approved nor subjected to any manufacturing oversight by the Food and Drug Administration, so they don't undergo the rigorous clinical trials that are required of meds made by commercial pharmaceutical companies. In the United States, asserts a 2017 review in the journal *Climacteric*, custom-compounded bioidentical hormone therapy "has become an unregulated drug manufacturer industry in disguise, without proper control and making false claims and misleading advertisements." And a 2020 report issued by the National Academies of Sciences, Engineering, and Medicine concluded that the lack of standardization can increase the possibility of overdosing, underdosing, or contamination. As NAMS points out on its website, custom-compounded bioidentical hormones may not even contain the prescribed amounts of hormones, "and that can be dangerous. For example, when the progesterone level is too low, you are not protected against endometrial (uterine) cancer. When estrogen levels are too high, there can be overstimulation of the endometrium and breast tissue, putting you at risk of endometrial cancer and possibly breast cancer."

Dr. DePree agrees. Bioidentical compounds are still drugs, she points out. "Don't equate 'bio' with something 'natural' and therefore risk-free," she says. "Taking any hormone involves some risk."

In 2013, *More* magazine did a now-famous investigation, obtaining twelve identical prescriptions for bioidentical hormone therapy (BHT) from a prominent ob-gyn who was concerned about the rampant use of unregulated hormones. The reporter had the prescriptions for Tri-Est (a combination of estradiol, estrone, and estriol, plus progesterone) filled at various compounding pharmacies across the country, then had the contents of the capsules analyzed by a lab. The results? Levels of estriol were subpotent, or lower than prescribed, while levels of the other two hormones were mostly superpotent, or higher than prescribed.

Nor are bioidentical custom-compounded hormones required to have any official labeling, so patients may be in the dark about some pretty vital information, such as warnings and contraindications. And without any explicit mention of risks, patients might be led to believe that there aren't any—one key reason why they might believe bioidentical hormone therapy is safer.

Pharmaceutical companies, meanwhile, are required to report complications from medications or serious and unexpected side effects directly to the FDA. And while compounded bioidenticals are marketed as more natural than commercial MHT formulations, they're still synthesized. Furthermore, as Dr. Lauren Streicher points out, compounding pharmacies don't manufacture hormones—they just *mix* them. Manufacturing factories, she says, sell the same active ingredients to both commercial pharmaceutical companies and compounding pharmacies. "It's the same stuff! It all comes from the same place!"

Compounding pharmacies can be useful for several reasons, such as if a person has allergies. For instance, if a drug contains peanut oil, a compounding pharmacy can eliminate the peanut oil for a patient with a peanut allergy so they can use the drug safely. If you do use a compounding pharmacy, make sure it's accredited by the Pharmacy Compounding Accreditation Board (achc.org), which has established quality and safety standards.

Many practitioners of bioidentical hormones will also recommend hormone testing—usually with saliva but also blood or urine—so their therapy can purportedly target specific hormonal problems. Not only is saliva testing unnecessary, asserts NAMS, but "it has also not been proven to be accurate or reliable." As I mentioned earlier, because hormone levels vary day to day as well as throughout the day, even a blood test, says NAMS, "cannot accurately reflect the body's hormone levels."

The appeal of saliva testing for doctors, says ob-gyn Lauren Streicher, "is that it gets people in the door regularly, and they spend a lot of money." She sighs. "Listen, I don't blame women who go to these people. We have ob-gyns and internists who know nothing about menopause, and women are desperate for help. Their own doctors aren't helping them, so of course they're going to go to people who say they will. And these prescribers are selling women misinformation, using all the right buzzwords, like 'natural,' and 'customized,' that are not only meaningless but completely misleading. It's been an issue of mine for a long time, along with a lot of other menopause experts."

This battery of lab tests, adds Wen Shen of Johns Hopkins, is not only unnecessary but often ridiculously expensive, because these tests are rarely covered by insurance. "I go by symptoms. If a patient is hot flashing through the night, I don't need to test her estrogen level to say, 'Yep, you're menopausal.'"

The American Medical Association, the American Society for Reproductive Medicine, and the Endocrine Society are among the many medical organizations that have cautioned against using compounded hormone therapy. Ultimately, the "bioidentical" label is a marketing distinction rather than one rooted in evidence, since many FDA-approved brand-name hormones not only meet the definition of bioidentical, says Shen, but are derived from natural sources, too, such as soy and yams. "Compounding pharmacies often get their ingredients from the same sources that Big Pharma does," says Shen. "I ask patients, 'Where do you think the pharmaceutical is getting the estradiol from?' The same plant sources. The same yams from Mexico. These ones are just well tested for safety and effectiveness."

DePree concurs. Many familiar brands of hormonal rings, creams, pills, and gels, she says, are both commercially manufactured and bioidentical—among them Estrace, Femring, Vivelle, Vagifem, Bijuva, and Prometrium. "And you know what you're getting with these products," she says.

Testosterone therapy, usually used to boost sexual function, is popularly prescribed to compounding pharmacies as well, because it's not FDA-regulated. Often, explains Streicher, it's in the form of a hormone pellet inserted under the skin of the hip that releases estrogen and testosterone over the course of six months. When a woman initially gets a pellet, she always feels great, says Streicher, "thanks to a huge surge of estrogen and testosterone that provides a supercharged libido, no flashes, and tons of energy."

But testosterone pellets, Streicher goes on, "generally have sky-high doses of estrogen and testosterone, well above what any women would produce at any time of her life."

Seattle-based author Emily Lynn Paulson had a radical hysterectomy and the removal of one ovary as part of her cancer treatment. When she experienced symptoms of menopause and sensed it might be imminent, her doctor suggested she see a hormone specialist.

"I should have sought out an endocrinologist, but instead, googled 'hormones' and the name of my town," says Paulson. "That brought me to a clinic that seemed to specialize in hormones."

The doctor Paulson saw recommended bioidentical testosterone pellets.

"She told me how low-risk and 'natural' the pellets are, and that they were basically a magical solution," she recalls. "I wasn't told any risks, other than 'some people get acne and a little increase in facial hair, but it's really rare.' What did I have to lose?" After her first insertion, Paulson noticed that she did indeed have more energy and a noticeable libido kick. But five months in, she started to feel worse. "I was anxious, my hair started falling out around my temples, my formerly smooth legs and armpits became furrier than ever, and I started getting acne on my back. Now I'm waiting for a referral to an endocrinologist."

• • • •

In the spring of 2022, the UK faced an acute shortage of MHT products. An estimated one million women in the UK, according to the National Institute for Health and Care Excellence, take MHT products—a sizable group, given that the total number of females is around 33 million. The National Health Service data shows that prescriptions have more than doubled over the past five years, thanks to a successful awareness campaign that I'll get to in an upcoming chapter. (In Scotland and Wales, MHT is actually free.)

When MHT supplies ran low in the UK, women became frantic, driving hundreds of miles in search of supplies, turning to the black market or other countries ("Shortages of HRT may force women to become drug mules by travelling overseas to buy vital supplies of medication," blared one headline). One woman called thirty pharmacies.

Others were reduced to bartering. "Meeting in a car park to exchange a tub of expensive face cream for a bottle of estrogen gel might sound like the far-fetched plot of a comedy detective show," wrote British journalist and *Cracking the Menopause* author Mariella Frostrup in *The Daily Mail*. "But that is what a good friend of mine was forced to resort to. Unable to get hold of her normal prescription for HRT, she was desperate, and ended up putting out a call for help on Facebook. It turned out that a friend of a friend kindly offered to do an exchange."

Some women reported that they felt suicidal; others had to stop going to work. Protests grew until health secretary Sajid Javid finally appointed an MHT tsar, Madelaine McTernan, who led the country's COVID vaccine taskforce, to commandeer the shortage crisis and arrange for relief. Once women become devotees of MHT, it seems, it can be tough for them to do without.

Chapter 10

The Restoration

Coming Back to Yourself

I want to be clear that my message throughout this book is not "do what I did." Every person is different, every experience with menopause varies wildly, and what worked for me might not work for you. My point is simply that if you have symptoms that are pulling down your quality of life, you deserve to get them treated.

I know that all this information is a lot to take in, so here are the highlights.

Be Mindful of Internalizing What's Known As "Gendered Ageism"

When I'm mulling over an idea for a book, I do a lot of crowdsourcing—as I did one night at dinner with a few friends, at a plant-festooned vegan soul-food place in the East Village. While we wait for our entrees, I ask them what sort of image they would propose for a book cover.

"My mom always said that when you go through menopause, you're invisible," says my friend Sari. Two of us, Sari and Lyla, are in perimenopause, while Shawn and I are fully going without the flow. Sari brightens. "I know! You know that old movie *The Invisible Man*? Maybe it could be an invisible woman."

"I don't get it," says my friend Shawn. "What would the image be? Just a blank page? I'm not sure that's compelling."

"No," says Sari. "You remember how the invisible man wore a hat and glasses and then he wrapped his head in a gauzy bandage? Maybe the invisible woman could be wearing those square wraparound glasses that my grandma in Boca wears."

I tell them that I want to avoid depressing images such as sunsets, which used to be a mainstay on menopause supplements.

"Subtle," says Shawn with a snort. "I know! How about you do a book cover with a plum that's looking in the mirror and sees a prune? That's how my skin feels. I am so dried out."

"Would the plum have eyes?" Sari wonders. "How does the plum see its reflection?"

"Actually, I don't feel like a plum sometimes," says Shawn. "Yesterday at work, a twenty-two-year-old girl in my office asked me if there were cell phones when I was a kid." She looks aggrieved. "Bitch, I'm not Grandma Moses!"

"But we didn't have cell phones when we were kids," I say.

Shawn nods. "Okay, true."

"We all had tan phones with cords that hung in the kitchen," I say. "Am I right?" Everyone nods. "When I was a teenager, if someone important called"—I make air quotes for *important*—"then

I would stretch the phone cord from the kitchen to the hallway closet near our front door, get in, and shut the closet door."

"The phone cord was curly," says Shawn. "It was fun to wrap around your finger when you talked."

"I remember seeing Michael Douglas talking on a cell phone on the beach in a movie and it blew my mind," says Sari.

"*Wall Street,*" Lyla breaks in. "Me too. I couldn't believe you could talk to someone while you were walking along on the beach. I saw the movie again a few years ago to see if it held up. Have you seen how big that phone is that he uses? It's hilariously large. It looks like he's talking into a shoe box."

"What year was that?" Sari wonders and checks her phone. "Nineteen eighty-seven," she announces.

"My point is that the girl in my office sees me in a way I don't see myself," says Shawn. She shrugs. "Somehow I thought getting older would take longer."

We return to ideas for the book cover. Reading glasses? A portable fan?

Yes, the jokes were made with affection, but also a frisson of condescension. It was clear we were uncomfortable with the idea of menopause (I'm not *old*-old!), so we went straight for *The Golden Girls* imagery to place ourselves firmly outside that category.

"I have a crew of friends who are ten years older than me, and I remember having no empathy when they started having hot flashes," says Denise Pines of WisePause Wellness. Pines had assumed that her friends' flashes were "kind of like you're in Miami and it's hot out." When she had a hot flash for the first time herself, "I thought I was having a spontaneous human combustion moment like in a bad horror movie, where the brains are flying everywhere. I never felt like that in my entire life."

Pines called every one of her friends "and apologized for not having any empathy. They probably don't even remember I had that reaction, but I do."

In a 2008 study published in the journal *Health Care for Women International*, college students from the United States and Mexico were surveyed about their impressions of women in different stages of reproductive life. A woman with a young baby was defined by the students as "happy," while menopausal women were labeled as "irritable" and "old." Young women were found to be especially harsh in their assessments.

This is nothing new to women in midlife, who often fear that if they look "old," they'll be judged as doddering. When some women began to allow their hair to go gray during the COVID-19 lockdown, researchers studied the consequences in a 2022 study in the *Journal of Women & Aging*. Investigators asked the international group of women why they went gray in spite of the chance of being stigmatized as old. The researchers identified two oppositional themes: competence and authenticity. Despite wanting to avoid perceptions of "old, thus incompetent," the women "risked" gray hair in order to feel authentic.

Of course, even though one woman said she was "flying her natural flag," this choice didn't make them feel entirely free. God forbid! After the women went gray, wrote researchers, "there was an apparently taken-for-granted assumption that gray hair must be countered by greater attention to its style and cut, application of cosmetics, non-surgical procedures, and careful choice of clothes to mitigate its aging effect."

The women, in other words, took to strategies like bold lipstick in order to reassure others that they weren't going to slump forward into a doze during meetings. It's not about hair color (although if you want to talk about bias, try to think of the female equivalent

"I'm going through perimenopause at the moment. It's really frying my brain. It is really bizarre, but it is the most glorious invitation into a new season and chapter in my life. . . . I'm the sexiest I've ever been. And when I say that, I mean I feel the most myself. . . . I'm going to be sexy all over the place. Living my life with my juice."

–Tracee Ellis Ross

of "silver fox"). It's about the legitimate fear that they will be judged as less vibrant, less mentally sharp, less relevant.

My snickering jokes about visor hats needlessly devalued older women. Language matters. Let's support and uplift each other, by words and actions, on the path that all female-born people will take.

Biases against older women are not only toxic for society, they are bad for you. If you build up a pessimistic attitude toward menopause, research shows this may manifest as worse symptoms. In a 2010 review in the journal *Maturitas*, UK researchers found that in ten out of the thirteen studies that they examined, women who had more negative attitudes toward menopause also reported having more problems with menopausal symptoms. You don't have to be a sociologist to conclude that this makes sense.

The more you learn about menopause, the less mysterious and frightening it is. The more often you casually bring it up in conversation, the more quickly the stigma disappears, for you and everyone else. Menopause is not a disease! It's a life stage. If you're lucky enough to live for a long time, you may be postmenopausal for fully half of your life.

Tell Your Loved Ones Exactly What Is Going On

If you don't know much about menopause, even as it happens to you, it's likely that the people around you are even more clueless. In 2017, *Health* magazine produced a video in which they asked men about perimenopause and menopause. The guys, a genial, well-meaning group, tried their best. "Menopause is when you're ovulating?" hazarded one when asked to define it. "No, that's probably not right." Another guy put forth this definition of perimenopause: "Maybe you get menopause a second time? I don't know." A third offered his explanation of a hot flash: "A woman is on her period, and she just gets too exhausted?" Well, he's not entirely wrong with that one. Keeping your symptoms to yourself, out of shame or "not wanting to bother anyone," can take a big toll on your relationships. If those around you have no idea what is happening, how can they support you? At the very least, they'll know why you're melting down (in body and perhaps mind) and give you a wide berth.

Silence breeds misunderstandings and hurt feelings. If you start avoiding sex, says Makeba Williams of Washington University St. Louis, partners can assume it's their fault. If you have a crying jag in front of your kid, they may also take it personally and feel upset and confused. When you forgo that beach weekend with your friends because you're self-conscious about your new body shape, you miss an opportunity to connect with them and share your story.

"Just talk about it," says Williams, "so that all of this sort of social, emotional, interpersonal complexity doesn't develop because you *weren't* talking about what is an absolutely normal physiologic event." Spark the conversation with loved ones, advises Williams, by defining in simple terms what menopause is and how it can affect your body. Name your symptoms, describe how those symptoms make you feel, and then ask for what you need.

Use the clear language that a doctor uses. Your vulva is not a pink canoe. It is not a coin purse. It is not a hot pocket.

Here is the script that I used on my husband, Tom, to give you an idea of how it might go.

> *Tom? Can you put your phone down? Thank you. I have something to tell you. I've started the transition into menopause—when your hormones that control reproduction start to leave your body, your period ends, and you are no longer fertile. It's not some sort of illness. It's a natural life process that affects all women.*

Because these hormones, such as estrogen, are present in almost every part of your body, when they leave your system, your body and brain react in different ways.

Some women go through menopause without a problem, but others can get pretty severe symptoms, and they can affect everything from your skin to your weight to your moods. These symptoms can last a few months or up to ten years. Ah, I see the "ten years" bit got your attention. It's a lot, right?

I know I've talked about how I'm going through menopause, but I haven't been very specific about what is happening to me, and I apologize for that.

I've been getting hot flashes, which is a sudden feeling of heat that travels in a kind of wave over my upper body and makes me sweat and turn red. Hot flashes are the most common symptom of menopause. No one knows what causes them. I get them mostly at night, and they wake me up. They usually last a few minutes, and it feels like someone's aiming a hair dryer at the highest setting right at my chest.

Women in menopause tend to collect weight around their middle. This is why you've heard some creative combinations of swear words from me as I try, and fail, to stuff myself into jeans that used to fit.

I try to be body positive; you know that I won't allow a scale in our house. Yet I do feel a little dismayed by the changes in my shape. The other night, when I was lying on my side as I was talking to you in bed, I looked down and saw that my gut rested on the mattress. I know you truly don't even notice, and I love you for it. But I notice.

Estrogen loss affects your brain, so I sometimes feel moody and irritable, and my memory is getting fuzzy. You're probably aware that you've had to finish my sentences a lot more, and that I often ask if you've seen my reading glasses when they're sitting on top on my head.

I feel annoyed that my hot flashes wake me at night and break up my sleep. I feel frustrated that my memory is not as sharp as it was. I am upset that sex hurts, as if it's my "fault."

I would be grateful if you could be patient with me and remind yourself that what I'm going through is biological. When you see me getting riled up or looking discouraged, I'd love if you could ask me what I need.

Thank you. You can look at your phone now. I see your fingers twitching.

Customize your script as needed. For example, if you're talking to your teenage son, you could say, *Remember when your voice started changing, and you were constantly embarrassed and annoyed because your body seemed to be going haywire and you had little control over it? That's what menopause feels like to me.*

"You can say to your teenager, 'Your body's changing, and you know what? My body is going to change, too,'" says Williams. "That will start the conversation. My son and daughter know what menopause is, because I don't feel the need to shield them from what it is."

A few weeks before my phone chat with Williams, she had been invited, she tells me, to speak in front of her child's fourth-grade class about reproductive health. "I told them, 'You know, you're going to go through puberty. And then at some point, your ovaries aren't going to work anymore, and we call that menopause. I talk about the whole spectrum of reproductive health.'"

When I hear this—a doctor who is doing her part to normalize this life transition, one fourth-grade classroom at a time—I am suddenly so moved that I choke up on the phone.

Don't Cover Up, Minimize, or Deny

Now when I catch myself concealing what's happening with my body or suppressing how I'm feeling, I train myself to be up front about it. Here's a perfect example: One afternoon, pre–vaginal estrogen, Tom and I were returning from a trip to the hardware store. As we pulled into the driveway and got out of the car, I suddenly had to get to the bathroom. I knew I had roughly ninety seconds before I started peein' m'pants, so I dashed to the front door, which was locked.

I implored Tom, who had the keys, to hurry. But at that point, he didn't know that this meant a gusher would appear within thirty seconds—because I had never told him about my new problem. He assumed I still possessed a competent bladder.

He ambled up the walkway, whistling, while I waited with my legs crossed. In twenty seconds, it would literally be Go Time.

Ten seconds. "Throw! Me! The! Motherfucking! Keys!" I screamed, in earshot of several neighbors doing yardwork (and who, I'm sure, suddenly went flamingo-still, gleefully hoping to hear more drama).

I ran over to Tom, snatched the keys, sprinted toward a bathroom—and in the midst of yanking down my pants, peed, like a new puppy, all over the bathroom floor. Later, I realized that because I was mum about the whole subject and, not for the first time, covertly cleaned up the mess, Tom had no inkling that I had menopausal bladder issues.

"Urge incontinence" is perhaps not the sexiest topic, unless you're into urophilia. But it had to be addressed.

I tried to be as direct and clear as possible. "I'm sorry I overreacted,"

I told him. "When estrogen leaves your body, the lining of your urethra, the tube that empties pee from your bladder, gets thinner and weaker, and your pelvic floor, the muscles that support your urethra, can also get weaker, so it doesn't work as well. It's very common among women. That's also why sometimes I pee when I sneeze, which is called, by those in the know, *peezing*. That's why I'm always tense when we go from the driveway to the house. Maybe, I don't know, we can turn it into a fun race or something."

I made myself be candid with him after I had a hair meltdown, too, when I was taking an author photo for this book. Author photos are arranged at least a year before publication, and I had yet to discover the wonder and magic of minoxidil. Tom did a photographic session with me outside in our backyard, where I tried to look authoritative, yet approachable.

When I saw the photos he took, my heart sank. The pattern on top of my head was the decimated Charlie Brown Christmas tree that Dr. Alison Bruce had described, and shiny patches of scalp were showing through.

I kept asking Tom to try again, while furtively arranging—or, in my sister Heather's words, *foofing*—my hair over the bald spots. Some two hundred rejected photos later, I finally confessed that my thinning hair was upsetting me.

"Why didn't you tell me?" he said. Off we went to the drugstore, where I bought some brown-tinted root cover. As I blasted away on the bald spots, I was reminded of the nineties infomercial for canned hair from TV pitchman Ron Popeil. (Who can forget the ad for the GLH System, or Great Looking Hair, in which one balding dude with a spectacular mullet gets his shiny pate sprayed and confidently announces "the babes are back"?)

But I did feel much better, and we got the picture.

Do Not—Repeat, Do Not—Randomly Google Your Symptoms

The internet, says New York City ob-gyn Kameelah Phillips, can undoubtedly be a useful resource—but perhaps not when you type "menopause" into Google. "When you do, you're going to get the sites that are quacky, that pay to be at the top of the Google search," she says. "Or if you literally google all of your symptoms, inevitably you're going to have cancer, right?"

Instead, Phillips recommends physician-vetted or physician-run websites, which I list in the Resources section at the end of the book. "If you don't have access to someone who specializes in menopause, these websites can serve as a proxy," she says. "They're evidence-based, they're written at a very easy-to-understand reading level that allows people to digest information and understand what their options are, and they're not going to scare the crap out of you."

As an experiment after chatting with Dr. Phillips, I consulted Dr. Google on three common symptoms of menopause.

Let's type in "memory lapses." Ah: up pops *The Cruelest Disease: Frontotemporal Dementia* and *When to Worry About Dementia*. (How about now?)

How about "night sweats"? Oh my: it could be cancer, an inflammation of the heart valve, a "mediastinal mass," or the title of a 2019 movie in which a "skateboarder investigates the mysterious death of his roommate." All sound frightful.

Let's move on to "irregular periods": *Irregular periods linked to a greater risk of an early death.* With that, the crap is officially scared out of me, and I close my computer.

Your Usual Beauty Routine Will Likely Fall Apart

One menopausal morning, I woke up and none of my go-to skin products worked anymore. Instead, they sat on top of my newly desiccated skin. My usual shampoo suddenly made my frizzy hair worse.

Remember: It's not the products; it's the latest iteration of your skin and hair.

My regimen required a complete overhaul. After much trial and error, I have landed on a cocktail of retinoids at night; peptides, amino acids, and sunscreen during every waking hour; and as a finisher, oils, oils, oils of every conceivable kind, which both moisturize my skin and lend it some luminosity. I use lip oil, hair oil, eyebrow oil, body oil, facial oil, and nail oil.

Now when I glance down at my arms, they almost resemble my fresh-skinned limbs of yore, thanks to the twin gifts of cheap olive oil and my hazy vision, courtesy of the steady degeneration of my eyes.

If you need help concocting a new skin-care routine, I recommend the social feed of two dermatologists, both affiliated with Mount Sinai Hospital in New York. They dispense clear advice and valuable tips for those of us in midlife. Dr. Rosemarie Ingleton (full disclosure: she is my derm) posts helpful videos on TikTok with humor and warmth (@ingletondermatology). Dr. Joshua Zeichner (I have visited him, too) has built a huge following on Instagram (@joshzeichnermd) for his straightforward, easy-to-grasp clips on subjects such as how to build collagen in your skin, dealing with adult acne, and how to prevent hair loss.

I also love the product tutorials and reviews from UK aesthetician and beauty industry expert Caroline Hirons on Instagram (@carolinehirons.) She's in her fifties (in one post, she attributes her glow to "menopause, and the tears of my enemies"), has a low tolerance for marketing hype, and is hilariously opinionated. ("Oh, that smells like ass," she says after cautiously sniffing an eye cream in one clip, then makes a gagging noise.)

And happily, marketers have woken up to the fact that women in menopause have hyper-specific skin needs. Ulta, the nation's largest beauty retailer, started carrying a menopausal skin-care brand, Womaness, for the first time in 2022. (As of this writing, it's just the one brand, but baby steps.)

Aside from Womaness, brands for menopausal skin, many formulated by dermatologists, are proliferating madly, among them SeeMe, PRAI Beauty, Korres's Meno-Reverse line, Emepelle, Caire Beauty, and Pause Well-Aging.

Get Moving—Which Does Not Have to Mean Training for a Marathon

Like it or not, many chronic diseases of aging start after menopause, so this is an opportune time to take stock of your health and craft a plan for the next chapter.

An easy way to stave off numerous ailments is simply to get moving. That said, it's tough for many of us to do. A 2018 SWAN study showed that only 7.2 percent of women transitioning to menopause are meeting the latest physical activity guidelines from the U.S. Department of Health and Human Services.

Which is not altogether surprising. If you're taking care of other people, older or younger, perhaps holding down a job, and don't have the energy that you once did, it's easy to put exercise aside.

But as mentioned, the guidelines are 150 to 300 minutes of moderately intense aerobic activities a week, which can be brisk walking, recreational bike riding, or yardwork. At the low end, 150 minutes is half an hour a day, five days a week—enough to fit in a semi-vigorous jaunt around the neighborhood.

The Endocrine Society's website warns that menopause speeds bone loss when estrogen levels drop (as mentioned, up to 20 percent of bone loss, in fact, can happen during this stage) and increases the risk of osteoporosis. Strength training both builds muscle back up *and* builds bone density—even in people who have reached the half-century mark.

A 2010 meta-analysis in the journal *Medicine & Science in Sports & Exercise* found that adults over fifty who lift weights can reverse age-related muscle loss. Strength training (or even weight-bearing aerobic exercises like walking or running) puts stress on bones that prompts bone-forming cells to make more—so they're stronger. The simple act of jumping up and down can even build bone, found researchers at Brigham Young University in 2004. They had premenopausal women do the following twice a day for four months: stand up, then jump into the air. When you land, wait for 30 seconds. Repeat twenty times. Easy! After the four months, the women's bone mineral density in their hips had improved significantly.

A friend of a friend named Carmen took up weightlifting in her forties and is an enthusiastic convert. A self-described "unathletic former benchwarmer," she now finds that lifting three times a week "is a consistent and reliable way to show up for my body," she says. "I love watching my numbers grow steadily over time. And now that I'm in perimenopause, I've found that the lifting is really helpful for managing my moods—my irritation sparks quick and hot these days, but lifting is a great outlet for recentering myself."

Carmen now delights in feeling strong. "I'm in awe of what my body can do, how it can change," she says. "I like the way my shoulders are sculpted from lifting, the way I no longer worry about getting my overhead luggage into the bin on planes, the confidence it gives me. I'm taking care of my body now, in the hopes it will take care of me as I continue to age."

As for me, I love my new swimming regimen at the Y. Being in the water makes me feel free. It feels like play. It was my favorite thing to do as a kid, and I've come full circle.

Again, whether I head out on a long walk or to the pool, I sell this to myself as movement—as in "I need to move." Or I'll jump up and mutter, "I need to clear my head," which makes me feel kind of like an action hero with the weight of saving the world on my shoulders. I know: I have a rich (or perhaps sad) fantasy life. Whatever works.

There's Menopause Support Outside the Doctor's Office

The more you share and compare what is going on with your transition, the better you will feel. There are all kinds of safe spaces for menopausal women to connect, from Facebook groups to online forums to community groups to apps. (And sometimes, as I did at the Menopause Café, it's often easier to share your symptoms with strangers.)

In many communities, points out Phillips, "the church is a really trusted resource for information and education. I'll tell you, I do talks for women's groups in churches all the time, for free—like, you're not gonna charge God, right?" She laughs. Inevitably, she says, the women in the group will ask her about their own symptoms, "so they get a talk *and* free consults!"

"Menopause has been a taboo subject for far too long. Why is it no one talks about it? It's past due time to fully embrace that women's bodies are not embarrassing, taboo, or a threat."

—Brooke Shields

Spaces like churches are helpful, Phillips says, "because it's an hour in a protected environment where people feel comfortable to share."

A menopause support group can pop up anywhere.

In 2022, a group even sprang up at the Kingfisher, an English pub in Ipswich owned by a mother and daughter who both struggled to get menopause support.

My friend Laura attends a book group with a bunch of women in their forties and fifties. When they noticed an increase in menopause chitchat before discussion of the book du jour, they decided to add an extra half hour before the book club "officially" started, just in case anyone wanted to show up early and swap tips. "They all did," she tells me. "Now we devote half an hour and get it out of our systems. I'm in perimenopause, so I love this part. Plus, half the time I haven't gotten around to reading the book, anyway."

Be Mindful That One Treatment Can Sometimes Address Multiple Symptoms

Several menopausal symptoms may be intertwined, as Dr. Nanette Santoro wrote in the *Journal of Women's Health*. Hot flashes may worsen sleep, which could then contribute to depressive symptoms. It therefore makes sense, she goes on, to consider single agents that can take care of more than one symptom.

Women with hot flashes and depression, for example, can be treated with hormone therapy if the depression is mild to moderate, or an SSRI. Those with hypertension and vasomotor symptoms, she writes, may be treated with the antihypertensive drug clonidine for both problems. If you're plagued by many different menopausal symptoms, raise this possibility with your doctor.

If You Are Able, See a Menopause Specialist

Ten minutes tacked onto your annual ob-gyn visit is not enough time to tackle a subject that can be as complex as menopause. "We have research study after research study saying that we as gynecologists and healthcare providers do a very poor job of asking about things like genitourinary symptoms of menopause and sexual health," says Dr. Makeba Williams. "So if we don't ask, we know that our patients don't bring it up. We need to give this time period in your life the attention it deserves."

You can find a certified menopause practitioner on NAMS's website. One or two visits may be all that's needed, says Williams. "For the majority of patients, I'm going to see them for a consultation, and they can be referred back to their primary provider for ongoing care." If patients are on hormone therapy or another medication, she adds, there may be one or two associated follow-ups. Many of these certified menopause practitioners are brilliant researchers at the pinnacle of their fields, with CVs as long as the King James Bible—and they'll be concentrating all their knowledge on *you*. Many have been quoted in this very book.

Let's say you live in southern Connecticut and type your zip code into NAMS's "Find a Menopause Practitioner" feature. Here we have, among other eminent experts, Lubna Pal, MBBS, FACOG, MS. Dr. Pal, whom I have quoted here and who is accepting new patients, is a professor of obstetrics, gynecology, and reproductive sciences; vice chair for education, obstetrics, gynecology, and reproductive sciences; and director of the Menopause Program at Yale Medicine. Her reams of scientific research include studies such as "Cardiometabolic Measures and Cognition in Early Menopause," "Effects of Oral vs. Transdermal Estrogen Therapy on Sexual

Function in Early Postmenopause," "Increased Incident Hip Fractures in Postmenopausal Women with Moderate-to-Severe Pelvic Organ Prolapse," and "Managing Menopause by Combining Evidence with Clinical Judgment."

This is the person who would take charge of your menopause care.

A certified menopause practitioner can deftly coordinate the many specialists that may contribute to your treatment, says Rachel Rubin of Georgetown. "Because it's not just one person who fixes all of your menopause problems, right?" she says. "You've got painful sex. You've got a bladder that's not working properly. You've got hot flashes. You're not sleeping. Your bones are becoming brittle. There are all of these problems, but they're all happening because of the exact same reason."

Wen Shen of Johns Hopkins, a board member of the North American Menopause Society, walks me through a typical consultation with her. She will begin by taking an extensive medical history and will do a gynecological exam if needed. "I go over a woman's personal medical history in great detail," she says, "because we know that there are issues that happen during a woman's pregnancy, like preeclampsia, or infertility issues or PCOS, or medical issues like diabetes or early menopause, that can portend quite a bit to her future cardiovascular health."

Next, she tunnels into the patient's social history—smoking, alcohol, activity level—before moving on to symptoms. Shen listens carefully and asks many, many questions. She sorts out which symptoms are related to menopause and which may be related to the natural process of aging.

She then develops a detailed treatment plan, which may include clinically tested remedies such as hormone therapy, nonhormonal therapies like SSRIs, and integrative remedies like acupuncture.

Mental health is covered, too, and she may refer patients to a psychiatrist or a sex therapist.

An expert, adds Lubna Pal of Yale Medicine, will home in on parts of your personal and family histories that may be particularly relevant to your own well-being—of which you may not even be aware. "For example, 'What was the age that you started having your periods? Did you have erratic periods during your reproductive years? Did you have an eating disorder at any stage of your life? Did you ever experience a bone fracture? Do you have any elderly family members who are 'stooping down' with advancing age, which likely reflects underlying osteoporotic fracture of spine?'"

All are relevant, Pal says, for your own bone health and your lifetime risk for fragility fractures. "I consider our bone mass or density as one of our retirement accounts," explains Pal. "If you were stingy with savings during your earning years, when reproductive hormones were plenty, your savings are likely light as you 'retire,' or enter menopause." In which case, she says, "your risk of developing osteoporosis and of sustaining a fracture in the postmenopausal years will be greater than someone else your own age who has more robust reserves in her account when she 'retires.'" If this is the case with your own history, she goes on, "we should be particularly vigilant about optimizing your bone health through simple strategies such as regular weight-bearing exercise and eating right. Also, now would not be the time to take up smoking."

Dr. Shen ensures that patients have adequate intake of dietary calcium and vitamin D_3, which helps bones absorb calcium. "One in two postmenopausal women will have an osteoporosis-related fracture in their lifetimes," she says. "These so-called fragility fractures don't heal properly because of decreased blood flow to the bones. People think, *Oh, osteoporosis, so I shrink an inch or two—no big deal.* Well, it is a big deal, because evidence shows that 80 percent of patients do not resume their previous level of function after a fragility fracture."

Doesn't it sound like heaven to have a highly trained expert carefully listen to your symptoms, understand perfectly what you are going through, and give you a plan so that you know exactly what to do?

"If you're desperate and your symptoms are getting worse and worse and your life is a mess, don't let a doctor tell you, 'Too bad, everybody goes through it, suck it up,' or 'It's all in your head,'" says Shen. "I can't make things perfect, but I can put the patient back to where they were, where they can cope with their lives again."

As I've said before, even if you can't see a menopause specialist, if your doctor is saying, "Too bad, everybody goes through it, suck it up," then it's time to find another doctor—one who hears you.

Conclusion

Meno-Positivity!

Recognize. Mobilize. Normalize.

One October evening in 1937, forty-five-year-old Byrdie Hollis and her husband stopped by the Rayville Drug Company in Rayville, Louisiana, for a bottle of Coca-Cola. As Mrs. Hollis began to drink, she felt what was later described as "some solid foreign substance" in her mouth, which she spat back into the bottle. The contents of the bottle were poured into a serving tray and examined. It was found, in that same description, "to contain dregs and also a decomposed and thoroughly soaked spider of the black widow specie."

After quaffing Eau De Spider and becoming ill, Hollis, quite understandably, lawyered up. When she sued for pain, discomfort, and injury, the soft drink company's defense was that her subsequent nausea, vomiting, abdominal pain, and nervousness was instead due to "the experience of her menopause."

Fortunately, the judge didn't buy it, and she was awarded $600.

But this was not the first, or last, instance of the so-called menopause defense. The story of how menopause was used as a legal defense to regularly gaslight women in the twentieth century, as told in the pages of the *Indiana Law Review*, is grimly fascinating. The "menopause defense" was used, writes Widener University law professor Phyllis T. Bookspan, "in male dominated courtrooms, as a bold and accepted means to devalue women's injuries, damages, and life worth."

It was hauled out when Anna Laskowski was knocked down and run over by a runaway horse and ice wagon in 1915 in Wayne County, Michigan. Laskowski's chest was crushed, her collarbones and two ribs were broken, and her shoulder was dislocated. The physician who examined her at the scene said he "found her nearly dead." When she sued People's Ice for injury, pain, and a chronic nervous condition called traumatic neurasthenia, People's Ice argued that her injuries were "practically repaired" and her nervous condition "resulted from the menopause."

The essential premise of the menopause defense, Bookspan continues, was that a woman approaching midlife "was either mentally ill, physically ill, or both." In essence, anything negative that could happen to a woman was already happening and couldn't be blamed on some faulty consumer good or careless driver who mowed over her.

The "menopause defense" finally ceased, writes Bookspan, in 1980—*not* because it was sexist or ageist, but because that year, the American Psychiatric Association dropped a diagnostic label called involutional melancholia (that was long given to the body of symptoms commonly associated with menopause) from its *Diagnostic and Statistical Manual*. "Without the benefit of easily admissible medical testimony about the emotional and psychological ills of

"Menopause is an age of opportunity—I think almost like a second adolescence."

—Cynthia Nixon

menopause," Bookspan writes, "the defense essentially disappeared from the legal scene."

What has remained is this: As long as we keep the subject of menopause in the shadows, we allow others to define it for us.

Recognize

Fortunately, more and more, we are dragging the subject of menopause into the light—and the momentum is only growing. Progress may be slow, but we are moving in one direction, and that is forward.

The UK is unequivocally leading the way in meno-friendly policies and initiatives. In 2022, for instance, the UK created a four-nation Menopause Taskforce to strategize ways that menopause support and services can be improved in education, physician training, and the workplace. Pink-haired firebrand and taskforce co-chair Carolyn Harris, a Welsh member of Parliament and Labour Party member, was successful in changing the law in Wales, Scotland, and Northern Ireland, thus removing the prescription fee for MHT, and is advocating to do the same in England. "It amazes me that the UK is seen as a world leader in this field as we still don't have this right yet—although I am determined to keep pushing until we do," she says. Children are learning about menopause in England's schools, too: the subject of menopause has been included on the Relationships and Sex Education (RSE) and Health Education curriculum since 2020.

Then there's the UK's Menopause Workplace Pledge, begun by the organization Wellbeing of Women in 2021 when organizers became concerned by the deluge of women leaving the workplace because of menopausal symptoms. A 2022 survey by the UK's Fawcett Society, a charity that fights for women's rights, found that 41 percent of women said they've seen menopause treated as a joke by people at work (a figure that roughly tracks the mention of menopause on the social media network Twitter, by my own rough survey).

The Menopause Workplace Pledge calls on employers to support colleagues going through menopause in the workplace and to talk "openly, positively and respectfully" about it. More than a thousand organizations have signed the pledge—and not small companies, either: they include the nation's Civil Service, the Royal Mail, and supermarket giant Tesco.

"The fear of being judged, considered past your best, incapable, or untrustworthy because of the impact of symptoms is very real for a lot of women," says Harris. "Employers being open about their support makes it so much easier for women to ask without fear of negative reactions or repercussions."

In 2022, London's mayor Sadiq Khan announced a groundbreaking menopause workplace policy for City Hall staff to dispel "one of the last taboos of occupational health." It included menopause leave, flexible hours for women with symptoms, temperature-controlled areas, training for managers, time off for medical appointments, and a campaign for greater awareness of symptoms. "What we've got to do as blokes, as managers, is talk about this, and to get rid of the stigma," Khan told the network ITV. "What I don't want is talented staff feeling embarrassed to talk about it. *You* shouldn't be embarrassed that I'm embarrassed."

As awareness of discrimination grows, women in the UK are seeking legal recourse. A 2022 report from the UK organization Menopause Experts finds that in the past two years, incidents of women filing menopause-related discrimination claims against employers have tripled. ("Support Menopause, or Prepare for Court, Firms Told," ran a 2021 headline in *The Times*.)

Firms are falling in line—and companies like the Nottingham-based organization Henpicked have sprung up to deploy a team of experts who work with businesses to make them menopause-friendly. When the businesses pass muster, they receive a Menopause Friendly accreditation, indicating that they have "created an environment where menopause can be talked about easily" and have put the right support in place for colleagues.

Other countries are stepping up as well. In Australia, more than $40 million was awarded in 2022 by the national government to establish specialist and service hubs for menopause, as well as an extensive education campaign for doctors and employers. "I know how debilitating it can be, how difficult it can be," Minister for Women Bronnie Taylor told *The Sydney Morning Herald*. She went through the transition herself and recalls "sitting around a board table and being so hot you want to open every window. If you say 'menopause' in a room full of blokes, they almost recoil. They don't know what to say. It doesn't tend to be talked about in workplaces."

How I wish every company established a Menopause Leave, as the Australian company Future Super did in 2021. Employees of the company (which provides investment services for Australia's retirement savings system, known as the "super fund") can take up to six days of paid leave a year—separate from sick leave—without needing a medical certificate. It's a small step forward, but it's a start.

Mobilize

The natural functions of a woman's body are often perceived as a liability in the workplace. As a 2019 editorial in the *Journal of*

Management posited, the three taboo Ms in working women's lives are menstruation, menopause, and maternity. "*What the fuck is she doing?*" I remember one guy hissing in my office upon hearing the sounds of my coworker's breast pump behind her closed office door.

Given the rising attention to pregnancy discrimination and breastfeeding policies in the United States, argues the editorial, the time is ripe to address the menopausal M—such as ensuring, at the very least, that employees have control over the temperature or air regulation in offices (i.e., small fans or opening windows).

You'd think that, if nothing else, companies would become more menopause-friendly in order to help their bottom line. It's been estimated in *Bloomberg* that global productivity losses tied to difficulties coping with menopause symptoms at work could amount to $150 billion per year.

In the United States, women make up nearly half of the workforce—a full 47 percent, according to government statistics. "And 44 percent of women in the workforce are older than forty-five," points out Wen Shen of Johns Hopkins. "1.3 million women transition into menopause annually in the U.S." Policymakers, adds Shen, "need to make menopause medicine into a public health priority." Yet most employees refuse to acknowledge menopause as a biological reality, let alone offer support for workers who are in the thick of it.

What can we do? The U.S.-based Let's Talk Menopause awareness campaign suggests that menopausal women create an employee resource group, or ERG. Also known as affinity groups, ERGs are voluntary, staff-led bands of employees with similar characteristics, among them ethnicity, gender, or personal identity. ERGs can be organized around women, veterans, LGBTQIA+, and disabilities, among others.

As workplace diversity and inclusion programs are becoming more widespread, ERGs, as *The Wall Street Journal* has reported,

"I've heard menopause described as a time in your life when you get back to the first unselfconscious ways that you emotionally were when you were, like, ten, and you were fully in your weird self and didn't really care what anyone else thought of you. I'm sure that's not everyone's experience, but the idea that it could be, the hope that it could be, is something that really keeps me going. I've seen it happen."

—author Emily Gould

are on the rise. Since the start of 2020, around 35 percent of companies have added or enlarged their support for ERGs, according to a 2021 study of 423 organizations by LeanIn.Org and McKinsey; an estimated 90 percent of major employers in the United States have ERGs. Uniting with like-minded others to form an ERG—even if it's just a handful of you—can increase your influence as well as your negotiating power. (Carnegie Mellon University features a step-by-step guide on how to get started—the link is in the Resources.) As the saying goes, if you want to go fast, go it alone. If you want to go far, go together.

An ERG for people in menopause could form a taskforce to brainstorm on ways to create a meno-friendly culture—and invite managers to sit in. Here are some changes in the workplace that you could promote, courtesy of Let's Talk Menopause as well as UK-based human resource experts CIPD:

- Have people in the company learn the symptoms of menopause. ("Menopause can affect people's confidence and it can be very daunting talking to someone who has no knowledge/awareness of the menopause," as CIPD's website sensibly points out.)
- Appoint an executive as the (accountable) menopause point person.
- Provide heat-reducing accommodations such as fans, cold drinking water, and cool rooms (so that women do not have to furtively thrust their heads inside the company freezer, pretending to look for a microwaveable burrito.)
- Allow breaks more often, so women can run to the bathroom if they're having, for example, an epic perimenopausal bleed.
- Ask for flexible work hours, like a later start time if hot flashes and night sweats make an employee's sleep hellish.

- Ensure that any company uniforms accommodate hot flashes.
- Designate some quiet rooms away from workplace noise, which can dial up stress as well as exacerbate problems with focus.

As NAMS president Stephanie Faubion told *Fortune* magazine, "Menopause in the workplace is where pregnancy and lactation were 30 years ago." Employers, she added, "need to understand this is a normal occurrence, and supporting women through this transition is in everyone's best interest."

As Joseph F. Coughlin, founder of the AgeLab at the Massachusetts Institute of Technology told *Today*, "One of the greatest under-appreciated sources of innovation and new business may in fact be women over 50, with new ideas, lots of life ahead of them and with the verve to get it done." Older women, he said, also have more education than at any time in history.

One declaration I have heard repeatedly as I've interviewed healthcare professionals, executives, and marketers is that millennials who are now heading into perimenopause are not sucking it up as previous generations did. Rather, they are exceedingly vocal in advocating for workplace support. "Oh my god, millennials are a pain in the ass," one CEO told me with equal parts irritation and admiration.

While the needs of menopausal women are still largely ignored in the workplace, it's a different story with marketers, who are waking up to the fact that these women have a slew of problems, a dearth of solutions, and major spending power. The global menopause market is estimated to swell to $22 billion by 2028.

At long last, the inclusive beauty trend has broadened to menopause. In the past few years, an armada of companies, many of them female-founded start-ups, have unveiled products formulated specifically for us, from supplements to shampoo to cosmeceuticals (cosmetics that treat skin issues).

Some companies have made these products easier to find, too. The UK's leading pharmacy chain Boots debuted a Menopause Support Hub in 2021, featuring targeted products such as vaginal moisturizers, menopause vitamins, and hair-thickening treatments. Perhaps other companies will follow suit, given that menopause is hardly a niche category.

Marketers have also caught on that products made to alleviate menopausal symptoms do not need to feature the dreary design of the days of yore—dull earth-toned bottles with a smattering of dried leaves on the label (why not just feature a coffin?).

Instead, many of today's products are housed in unabashedly luxurious packaging, with hefty sculptural glass and gold lettering—a signal that they're to be proudly displayed, not stashed away in a drawer with the skin-tag removal cream and the hemorrhoid ointment. Often the word *menopause* is clearly inscribed on the label, too, a welcome alternative to vague, unpleasant phrases like *anti-aging.*

Veteran beauty executive Rochelle Weitzner told me that she founded the menopause skincare line Pause Well-Aging after going through perimenopause and asking herself, *Where the hell are the products for us?* Weitzner, the former CEO of the skincare company Erno Laszlo, realized that during a career spent promoting beauty as youthful radiance, "I'd not only neglected the millions of women older than me—I'd neglected my own future."

Even a few short years ago, before she founded the brand in 2019, Weitzner says it was a struggle to get it off the ground: convincing skittish investors to take the plunge took two years and two hundred pitches. After finally securing an investor, she met with people from beauty publications who balked at the idea, because, as she told me, they didn't want readers to—sigh—feel bad about themselves. Now celebrities are giving menopause a glamorous gloss by founding menopause brands. Gwyneth Paltrow, who once lamented that we don't have a great example of a menopausal aspirational woman in our society, seems to be stepping into that role. Paltrow and a group of celebrity investor friends, among them Cameron Diaz, Drew Barrymore, soccer star Abby Wambach, and author Glennon Doyle, have backed the telehealth start-up Evernow, which provides virtual direct-to-consumer hormone therapy for the perimenopausal and menopausal. A subscription includes unlimited access to its medical team and the delivery of well-priced hormone therapies estradiol or paroxetine, supplemented with progesterone when needed. Investors have scrambled to open their wallets. As of this writing, Evernow has raised over $28 million in funding.

Of course, one aspect of menopause care still in urgent need of disruption is delivering treatment and solutions into the hands of lower-income people, who, in many cases, need it most.

"There are these amazing companies coming forward that are really addressing menopausal care," says Laurie Zephyrin, clinical assistant professor of obstetrics and gynecology at NYU's Langone School of Medicine and vice president for advancing health equity at the Commonwealth Fund. "But, you know, people have to pay out of pocket, and they haven't figured out the insurance piece. So I would say for the innovators, how does one ensure that it can reach all people across the income stream?"

Menotech is a word that is increasingly popping up in business journals. In the biomedical world, several companies, among them New York–based Gameto, are raising big dollars to research delaying—or even eliminating—menopause. As the company website puts it, Gameto is "making the medical burden of menopause optional. When ovaries are termed 'geriatric' by many traditional medical criteria, the rest of the body is certainly not. Considering human healthspan and lifespan have increased significantly, we believe this biological phenomenon is no longer fit for purpose and is a problem worth solving."

Some would debate this idea, but at least it's now part of the conversation.

Biotech start-up Celmatix, meanwhile, is developing a drug that will delay menopause by fifteen years, in order to thwart the health issues that can arrive with it, such as heart disease. As CEO Piraye Beim told *Fortune* magazine, "menopause control is the real moonshot."

Until recently, menopause was one of the few women's life stages without much of a digital landscape. Community-building tools have since proliferated, from apps like Peanut Menopause, a division of the popular social network brand Peanut, which has a Tinder-like matching feature, to content platforms such as Menopause Made Modern, for people of color.

One of the most heartening developments is that ob-gyns like Kameelah Phillips have taken to social media—and have built up sizable followings of people who are eager for information on women's health. "I love that we're all learning so much, especially about health, through the internet and Instagram and TikTok," says Dr. Phillips. "It's definitely empowered women to speak out and realize that there's a community of people with a shared experience."

Today, in the U.S., the majority of ob-gyns are now female; in 2019, for the first time in history, more U.S. medical students were women than men; menopause will be part of their shared experience, too.

The subject of menopause continues to bubble up in the culture in smaller but noteworthy ways, where women in this transition are portrayed as having power. In Season 4 of the popular Danish political thriller *Borgen*, politician Birgitte Nyborg complains to her doctor: "I can't keep changing my shirt three times a day, I'm the foreign minister." The 2022 novel *The Change*, a revenge-fantasy thriller by Kirsten Miller that is being adapted for a TV series, tells the tale of former executive Jo Levison, whose "free-floating rage and hot flashes that arrive with the beginning of menopause feel like the very last straw—until she realizes she has the ability to channel them, and finally comes into her power." Would a plot about a woman harnessing the potent force of her hot flashes have sold a decade ago?

It's an encouraging sign that an emerging category of romance novels features women in menopause as part of the "Later in Life" genre—yes, women in midlife have sex!

"This genre is growing because there is a really strong desire for books with older heroines dealing with the issues of middle age," says paranormal romance fiction author Lisa Manifold, who went through menopause herself at forty-five. "I'm not a twenty-something woman anymore, and neither are many of my readers." Among the delightful titles in Manifold's six-book series The Oracle of Wynter are *Necromancy & Night Sweats*, *Hoodoo & Hair Loss*, *Incantations & Insomnia*, and *Hexes & Hot Flashes*.

You can now send menopause greeting cards, too, courtesy of popular illustrator Emily McDowell. One, a colorful block of type, reads: *Menopause! I have some questions. WTF? WTF?*

Normalize

This may be the most important element of bringing menopause into the light.

"Make connections, make friends, join communities, and really honor yourself. You're getting ready to make that transition to menopause, so pay attention to where you're at emotionally, physically, and mentally. The women who stress have it longer and harder, but the ones who accept it have it shorter, and less severe."

–Cameron Diaz

If more than a billion human beings will reach menopause by 2025, how can this many people continue to stay silent about it? We'll see real and lasting change when we start talking openly. Be that person who breaks the silence. Tell coworkers in a meeting to give you a minute because you're having a hot flash. Say this without cringing or apologizing. Inform your family about this life transition until they are sick of hearing about it and it has fully sunk in. Describe to your doctor in detail exactly what is happening in your body and mind. Ask friends if they're having symptoms and tell them what remedies have worked for you. The more we talk about it—to friends, family, coworkers, policymakers, your mail carrier—the more we steadily chip away the stigma.

"The best way to combat shame is to stare it in the face," advises psychologist Melissa Robinson-Brown of Mount Sinai. "Don't hide. Start with your family and close friends and share your experiences. You will likely initially experience discomfort, and that's okay. It will feel awkward, and you may stumble over your words. Embrace that discomfort. Notice it. But don't let it stop you."

The more you push through the uncomfortable feelings, says Robinson-Brown, the easier it will become. "And in turn, you will likely be helping those close to you feel more comfortable sharing their own experiences, too," she continues. "But in order to change the culture, we have to get comfortable with these discussions. Society has absolutely made up these rules, and the patriarchal, sexist nature of our society has created this sense of shame. It's up to us to change the narrative."

I am careful now to avoid turning any shame upon myself. I've become especially aware of the power of self-talk, and the way ageism slips into the dialogue I'm even having with *myself.* When I'm looking in the mirror, I resist with all my might the impulse to think, *Oh my, your neck resembles a Slim Jim* or *Wow, that's some frizzy-looking hair, you look like that ad for the Drew Barrymore movie* Firestarter *in the eighties.*

My friend Lisa told me she calls herself "sweetheart" when she's feeling anxious. ("You're going to be just fine, sweetheart.") I do the same. Lisa's college-age daughter loved this idea so much that she had *sweetheart* tattooed on her arm as a tribute to Mom.

Practicing self-compassion has been shown to yield all kinds of benefits, including lower levels of anxiety and depression. Rebecca Thurston of the University of Pittsburgh and her colleagues found, in a 2021 study, that middle-aged women who were more self-compassionate had a lower risk of developing underlying vascular disease. And who needs a little kindness during this transition more than you? Who deserves it more than you?

Along with speaking freely, casually, and often about menopause, arm yourself with information. Being perpetually baffled makes you feel powerless. The more you know about menopause, the calmer you will be. A 2020 study of middle-aged teachers in Eritrea in the journal *BMC Women's Health* found that when they were given a three-day course on menopause, their attitudes toward it significantly improved. When women's awareness increases, the researchers wrote, "it improves their attitude, health behavior, and health habits which eventually lead to an improvement in their quality of life." That's pretty significant.

Knowing that symptoms can be treated, or at least managed, dials down the fear and worry.

As Makeba Williams of Washington University St. Louis points out, after you enter menopause, "you remain in it as long as you are on this earth. And if you're going to spend a potential half of your lifetime in a particular stage, we, as doctors, want those to be some of the happiest and healthiest years for you. This is the stage in life when you've got the time back! You can be on top of this. You can thrive. You just need the right information."

One reason I viewed menopause with suspicion and dread *before* I went through it is that I didn't know much about it. I'm not alone. A 2010 Taiwanese study of women across the menopausal transition in *BMC Women's Health* found that the women with negative attitudes toward menopause were younger, while the postmenopausal women "had a more positive attitude once they actually faced menopause."

This has been my experience, too. This is a time, says Robinson-Brown, when "if you have kids, they may be older, meaning more independence for them and more free time for you. You may be more advanced in your career or starting a new career, which can also be exciting. It's a time to potentially travel, start new hobbies, go out more, reconnect with old friends." (Or make new friends: my sister Dinah told me she has vowed to make at least one new friend a year: "a real friend that I really connect with, not an acquaintance.")

Hadine Joffe of Harvard says that this time period is "an opportunity to reflect and say, 'You know, I'm at this juncture of midlife, what's meaningful to me? What's important to me?' As opposed to, 'Oh my gosh, I'm doomed.'"

If women who are not yet menopausal "could glimpse what this state of peaceful potency might be," wrote author Germaine Greer, "the difficulties of making the transition would be less."

Not long ago, I was scrolling through the comments in a *New York Times* story about menopause. One in particular resonated with me. "You know what?" wrote a person who called themselves Northern Light. "I enjoyed being in my body BEFORE estrogen took over and I developed breasts, a monthly period, and sexual urges that led sometimes to poor choices."

I did, too—although I am of the opinion that midlife does not magically confer the ability to make good choices. You'll notice that throughout this book, I have avoided asking you to embrace your "wisdom."

The word *wisdom* appears very, very often on menopause memes, and frankly, I feel like this puts a lot of pressure on us. What if we *don't* become wise? Life experience doesn't always translate to "wisdom." Just because you've reached midlife doesn't mean you're automatically qualified to retreat to the mountaintop to drop truth bombs on supplicants.

As Nora Ephron wrote in *I Feel Bad About My Neck*, "Every so often I read a book about age, and whoever's writing it says it's great to be old. It's great to be wise and sage and mellow. I can't stand people who say things like this."

But I do agree with *The New York Times* commenter on making fewer poor choices. I would much rather be in my fifties than in my twenties—and I had a wild time in my twenties. I was a reporter at *Rolling Stone* and a veejay on MTV2. When I wasn't interviewing famous musicians (which doesn't impress my teen, who will nonchalantly nail me with *Who's Bono?*), I was running around New York City, going to clubs and bars, being young and free.

I wouldn't go back to that time period for anything. My mind was never, ever at rest; it was in turmoil all the time. I made horrendous choice after horrendous choice, from substances I ingested to people I dated. I was obsessively preoccupied with what others thought of me and hustled constantly to please everyone but myself. I tell people in their twenties that I vastly prefer to be the age that I am, and they don't believe me. I wouldn't have believed this, either, when I was their age—but it happens to be true.

Adieu to periods and nonstop angst! I don't second-guess myself anymore. I know what I like. My mind is quiet. I am direct with others, which saves time and conserves mental and emotional energy. I surround myself with people who sustain and uplift me. Actress and activist Jameela Jamil disclosed something on her podcast *I Weigh* that has resonated with me. Jamil announced that she didn't have the "exhausting" impulse to win people over anymore. She said that when she has a new conversation with someone, she is no longer thinking, *Am I impressing them? Am I engaging them?*

"I'm looking for 'Are we connected? Is there any reason I should continue this conversation or pursue anything further with this person?'" said Jamil, who is in her thirties and arrived at this insight admirably early. "I think it's worrying when we walk around constantly auditioning for other people, and we're discouraged from thinking, 'What serves us?'"

Life is too short, Jamil goes on, "and I will not give a moment of my energy to someone who I actually don't wish to be close to. Not a single moment! I consider my time too valuable. I consider *myself* too valuable to have to put myself in that position." I think about her words a lot, and when I catch myself "auditioning," I will myself to stop.

I'm now ready to step fully into what author Alice Walker calls "a time of extremely high power and shapeshifting."

"This can truly be the best time in our lives," says Rochelle Weitzner, "when we have the most freedoms, and just don't give a crap what other people think of us." I love thinking of menopause as an era of freedom.

In her book *Revolution from Within*, Gloria Steinem wrote that menopause brought "a much longed-for era of relative peace and self-expression." That sounds right to me, too.

I hope that you will learn everything you can about menopause, share your experience with others, seek treatment if you need it, and refrain from freaking out.

My dream is that our view of menopause as an ordinary developmental passage eventually becomes so saturated in our culture, so thoroughly banal, that when it arrives, it's greeted with *Eh, it is what it is.*

My most fervent wish is that when people realize they are entering this natural, normal life stage, they react not with alarm or confusion, but with a shrug.

• Resources •

WEBSITES

The **North American Menopause Society** (menopause.org) offers easy-to-follow videos, FAQs, and a nationwide list of certified menopause practitioners.

The **International Menopause Society** (imsociety.org/for-women) is a leading global resource on the latest menopause research and has useful interviews, webinars, and podcasts.

The website **Red Hot Mamas** (redhotmamas.org) is an all-purpose and invaluable resource, with a Menopause A–Z guide, a newsletter, events, and survival tips. One of the website's most pleasing features is "Ask the Experts," where you can directly email your menopause question to a member of its advisory board of eminent experts.

The **University of Rochester Medical Center's menoPAUSE blog** (urmc.rochester.edu/ob-gyn/ur-medicine-menopause-and-womens-health/menopause-blog.aspx) features up-to-date advances on menopause management as well as thoughtful and incredibly detailed answers to readers' questions.

The **American College of Obstetricians and Gynecologists** (acog.org) offers evidence-based information on women's health.

The **Northwestern Center for Sexual Medicine and Menopause** (sexmedmenopause.nm.org), founded by Dr. Lauren Streicher, has plenty of detailed information and videos, as well as a link to Dr. Streicher's funny, solution-driven podcast, *Dr. Streicher's Inside Information: THE Menopause Podcast.*

The **National Center for Complementary and Integrative Health** (nccih.nih.gov) offers the latest research and safety information on herbs, supplements, and alternative therapies.

The **American Urogynecologic Society** (augs.org) has a useful "Find a Provider" feature; just type in your location.

The **Study of Women's Health Across the Nation** (swanstudy.org) issues frequent updates on their ongoing menopause research.

The **Society for Women's Health Research** (swhr.org) offers a downloadable "Menopause Preparedness Toolkit: A Woman's Empowerment Guide" that includes wellness tips and a menopause-care journal.

Omisade Burney-Scott's ***Black Girl's Guide to Surviving Menopause*** podcast is for Black women negotiating the different stages of menopause, "along with their ever-evolving identities, relationships, careers, responsibilities, and societal tropes."

Only 6 percent of the physician workforce is Black, according to the Association of American Medical Colleges. Find a culturally sensitive doctor in your neighborhood on the website **BlackDoctor**; just plug in your zip code (blackdoctor.org.)

GoodRx (goodrx.com) finds the lowest prices for prescription drugs in your area and sends drug coupons to your phone that you can take to your pharmacist.

CostPlusDrugs (costplusdrugs.com) is a website that offers common medications at sharply discounted prices. Find your medication in their online store, sign up for an account, have your doctor send in the prescription, and the company delivers it straight to you.

The **Open Path Psychotherapy Collective** (openpathcollective.com) is a nonprofit nationwide network of mental health professionals who provide in-office mental health care at a steeply reduced rate.

The **American Psychoanalytic Association** (apsa.org) has a list of low-fee clinics across the country.

Carnegie Mellon University features a helpful printable toolkit on how to form an employee resource group (cmu.edu/hr/assets/erg/vp-erg-toolkit-2020.pdf).

Peanut Menopause (peanut-app.io/blog/menopause), a subset of the women's social network Peanut, is a free app that provides a space for menopausal women to meet and ask questions. Participants can even use the app's matchmaking feature to discover other women with whom they can chat live, using messaging or video.

The telehealth company **Alloy** (myalloy.com) has a network of menopause-trained doctors who will assess your symptoms and prescribe FDA-approved plant-based bioidentical hormones delivered straight to your door (no waiting for months to see a doctor).

The organization **Let's Talk Menopause** (letstalkmenopause.org) has downloadable posters with symptoms to spread awareness.

Similarly, the **Pausitivity** (pausitivity.co.uk) menopause awareness campaign, begun by two women in the UK, features a printable poster on their website with menopause symptoms for display not just in doctors' offices but in "workplaces, libraries, gyms, hospitals, or any public space." It's available in English, French, German, Dutch, and Urdu.

Several ob-gyns recommended the vaginal dilator company **Soul Source** (soulsource.com) for well-made silicone dilators created by a gynecologist and sex therapist.

The **Menopause Café** (menopausecafe.net) hosts discussions about menopause all over the world.

RELIABLE WEBSITES FOR HEALTH INFORMATION

Mayo Clinic (mayoclinic.com)

Cleveland Clinic (clevelandclinic.com)

MedlinePlus (medlineplus.gov)

National Institutes of Health (nih.gov)

Harvard Health Publishing, the consumer health education division of Harvard Medical School (health.harvard.edu)

RxList, a pharmacist-founded medical website that's part of the WedMD network, offers detailed pharmaceutical information about generic and brand drugs (rxlist.com)

SOCIAL MEDIA ACCOUNTS

Menopause doctor **Heather Hirsch**, who practices at Brigham & Women's Hospital in Boston, is adept at breaking down complicated medical information in a clear way. She has an outstanding YouTube channel, podcast (*Health By Heather Hirsch*) and Instagram account (@heatherhirschmd).

Ob-gyn **Kameelah Phillips** delivers science-backed tips with warmth and humor on her Instagram account @drkameelahsays.

Ob-gyn **Jen Gunter**, author of the instant classic *The Menopause Manifesto*, wields a "lasso of truth" on her Instagram account @drjengunter.

The Instagram account of yoga teacher and embodiment coach **Gabriella Espinosa** (@gabriellaespinosa) is filled with tons of useful information on how to "connect to your body's wisdom and own your power and pleasure through midlife and menopause."

Ob-gyn **Mary Jane Minkin**'s comprehensive website **Madame Ovary** (madameovary.com) and podcast, ***Lady Parts***, answers every menopause question under the sun.

Urologist and sexual medicine specialist **Maria Uloko** posts on Instagram at @mariaulokomd.

Urologist and sexual medicine specialist **Rachel Rubin** posts on Instagram at @drrachelrubin.

The **Queer Menopause Collective** offers menopause support and education for LGBTQIA+ folks on Instagram at @queermenopause.

The Facebook support groups **Perimenopause Hub** and **Perimenopause WTF?!** are closed, confidential communities where you can talk freely about symptoms and connect with others in a safe atmosphere—and nothing, I mean nothing, is off-limits.

Acknowledgments

Thank you, first and foremost, to the experts I have consulted and quoted in this book, and all the truly heroic people who are working to improve women's health. I must single out Dr. Mary Jane Minkin of the Yale School of Medicine, who was so generous with her time and knowledge when I was beginning the book.

I am so grateful to my agent, Alexandra Machinist, for her guidance, unerring instincts, and keen knowledge. She's the embodiment of the sort of dazzling, well-read, witty New Yorker I desperately hoped to meet when I came to the city as a rube decades ago. I've said many times that my life changed for the better when I met her. Thanks also to her delightful assistant, Mina Bozeman.

I am similarly grateful to Michelle Howry, who is all kinds of wonderful: kind, gifted, enthusiastic. Whenever I tell someone that she is my editor, the inevitable response is "Oh, I love her."

My deepest thanks to the outstanding Putnam team, all of whom have made this process a joy: Ashley Di Dio, Sally Kim, Alexis Welby, Ashley McClay, Molly Pieper, and Samantha Bryant.

Thank you to the hardworking publicists Ashley Hewlett and Kristen Bianco.

Production team, I appreciate you so very much: Emily Mileham, Maija Baldauf, Claire Winecoff, Fabiana Van Arsdell, and Tiffany Estreicher. Nancy Inglis is a splendid copy editor whose diligence—and wit—made the book's final stretch a pleasure.

Thanks also to Jessica Grose, Melonyce McAfee, Lori Leibovich, and Farah Miller, my brilliant editors at *The New York Times,* who have inspired me in so many ways.

I am indebted to the unfailingly helpful and upbeat librarians at Madison Library in Madison, New Jersey, and to Mia Matos, who finessed my endnotes.

With every year that passes, I am more grateful for my friends, who shared their stories and provided incisive comments. Thank you to Faith Salie, Tina Exarhos, Judy McGrath, Susan Kaplow, Lauren Mechling, Menna Seleshi, and Tracy Chang. Extra special thanks to my beloved lifeline, Julie Klam.

Lifetime gratitude to Bob Love, Karen Johnston, Abigail Walch, Terry Real, Celia Ellenberg, Laura Tisdel, Vanessa Mobley, and Flora Stubbs.

I owe everything to my parents, Jay and Judy Dunn. When I decided to become an author at the age of eight, they set up a table at the end of our driveway to sell the "books" I had "written" (and told me not to give up when I was left with a sizable pile of remainders). They supported me, as they always do, throughout the writing of this book, and weathered countless panicky phone calls. The lessons they instilled in me about perseverance, resilience, and considering the perspectives of others have informed my work and my life. Mom and Dad also accept with good humor—or perhaps resignation—that I feature them in many of my books. What's a writer to do when they consistently deliver solid-gold quotes?

A huge thank-you to my sisters and lifelong pals, Dinah Dunn and Heather Stella. How can I possibly attempt to write how much they mean to me? How can I even try without crying?

I could not have completed this book without the help and encouragement of my husband, Tom Vanderbilt. Not only has he read countless drafts, but as he's learned about menopause, he has become my most thoughtful ally during my transition, ensuring that I get enough rest, prying me from my computer for long walks, soothing me during my vertiginous mood swings, and diligently replacing my bottle of hot flash spray when it runs out. Thank you, Tom.

• Notes •

CHAPTER 1: WHAT TO EXPECT WHEN YOU'RE NO LONGER EXPECTING

3. **Perimenopause lasts, on average, for four years:** "Perimenopause." Cleveland Clinic, last modified October 15, 2021; https://my.clevelandclinic.org/health/diseases/21608-perimenopause.

3. **it can stretch to eight:** "Menopause 101: A Primer for the Perimenopausal." North American Menopause Society, accessed July 8, 2022; https://www.menopause.org/for-women/menopauseflashes/menopause-symptoms-and-treatments/menopause-101-a-primer-for-the-perimenopausal.

3–4. **a *Love Boat* episode:** Mandi Bierly, "The Love Boat on DVD: Heaven or Hell?" *Entertainment Weekly,* October 27, 2008; https://ew.com/article/2008/10/27/the-love-boat-j/.

5. **"In my adult life":** Oprah Winfrey, "How Heart Palpitations Led Oprah to Discover She Was Approaching Menopause." Oprah.com, September 24, 2019; https://www.oprah.com/health_wellness/oprah-reveals-how-she-realized-she-was-approaching-menopause.

6. **studies have found, for women of color:** Brian D. Smedley, Adrienne Y. Stith, and Alan R. Nelson, eds., "Unequal Treatment: Confronting Racial and Ethnic Disparities in Health Care." National Library of Medicine, July 8, 2022; https://pubmed.ncbi.nlm.nih.gov/25032386/.
6. **those of larger size:** Jennifer A. Lee and Cat J. Pausé, "Stigma in Practice: Barriers to Health for Fat Women." *Frontiers in Psychology* 7, no. 2063 (2016): 2063; doi: 10.3389/fpsyg.2016.02063.
7. **A 2013 survey found that fewer than one in five:** Mindy S. Christianson et al., "Menopause Education: Needs Assessment of American Obstetrics and Gynecology Residents." *Menopause* 20, no. 11 (2013): 1120–25; doi: 10.1097/GME.0b013e31828ced7f.
7. **Not until 1993 were women and minorities:** Institute of Medicine, "NIH Revitalization Act of 1993 Public Law 103-43," in *Women and Health Research: Ethical and Legal Issues of Including Women in Clinical Studies,* Anna C. Mastroianni, Ruth Faden, and Daniel Federman, eds. (Washington, DC: National Academies Press, 1994), https://www.ncbi.nlm.nih.gov/books/NBK236531/.
8. **according to the nonprofit FAIR Health, the national average cost:** "Royal Birth Spotlights U.S. Childbirth Costs," Fair Health, June 28, 2018, https://www.fairhealth.org/article/royal-birth-spotlights-us-childbirth-costs.
8. **insurance claims from 500,000 women:** Karen N. Peart, "The High Cost of Hot Flashes in Menopause." Yale School of Medicine, August 27, 2014; https://medicine.yale.edu/news-article/the-high-cost-of-hot-flashes-in-menopause/.
9. **only 18 percent said they felt "very informed":** Colette Thayer and Cheryl Lampkin, "Perimenopause Is More Than Hot Flashes: What Women Need to Know." AARP, May 2021; https://www.aarp.org/research/topics/health/info-2021/perimenopause-hormonal-changes-impact.html.
9. **the multiple forms of menopausal urinary incontinence:** Sheela Nambiar, *Fit After 40: For a Healthier, Happier, Stronger You* (Hachette India, 2018).
11. **"it had ceased to be with Sarah":** Genesis 18:11 (Revised Standard Version).
11. **"moved of itself hither and thither":** Francis Adams, *The Extant Works of Aretaeus, The Cappadocian* (Boston: Milford House, 1972; originally published 1856); http://www.perseus.tufts.edu/hopper/text?doc=Perseus%3Atext%3A1999.01.0254%3Atext%3DSA%3Abook%3D2%3Achapter%3D11.
11. **Helen King wrote in *Hysteria Beyond Freud*:** Helen King, *Hysteria Beyond Freud* (Berkeley and Los Angeles: University of California Press, 1993), 19.
12. **Emily Martin unearthed this:** Emily Martin, *The Woman in the Body: A Cultural Analysis of Reproduction* (Boston: Beacon Press, 2001), 19.
12. **according to the authors of *The Curse: A Cultural History of Menstruation*:** Janice Delaney, Mary Jane Lupton, and Emily Toth, *The Curse: A Cultural History of Menstruation,* 2nd rev. ed. (Urbana: University of Illinois Press, 1988), 215.

12. **as Susan Mattern writes:** Susan P. Mattern, *The Slow Moon Climbs: The Science, Mystery, and Meaning of Menopause* (Princeton, NJ: Princeton University Press, 2019), 272.
13. **the 1897 book *The Menopause*:** Andrew F. Currier, *The Menopause; A Consideration of the Phenomena Which Occur to Women at the Close of the Child-Bearing Period* (New York: D. Appleton and Company, 1897), 280–81.
13. **Anxiety is one of the thirty-four various symptoms:** Lindsey Todd, "What Are the 34 Symptoms of Menopause?" Medical News Today, June 20, 2021; https://www.medicalnewstoday.com/articles/what-are-the-34-symptoms-of-menopause.
13. **Alexander Hubert Providence Leuf:** Alexander Hubert Providence Leuf, *Gynecology, Obstetrics, Menopause* (Philadelphia: Medical Council, 1902), 296–97.
13. **In the nineteenth century, writes health sciences professor:** Elizabeth Siegel Watkins, *The Estrogen Elixir: A History of Hormone Replacement Therapy in America* (Baltimore: Johns Hopkins University Press, 2010), 17.
14. **first hormonal product marketed for menopause, called Ovariin:** Thom Rooke, *The Quest for Cortisone* (East Lansing: Michigan State University Press, 2012), 31.
14. **Edward Doisy isolated estrogen in 1929:** Henrick Dam, "Edward A. Doisy: Biographical." The Nobel Prize, accessed July 8, 2022; https://www.nobelprize.org/prizes/medicine/1943/doisy/biographical/.
14. **My favorite Premarin ad:** *Psychiatric News* 10, no. 23 (December 3, 1975), 6.
14. **laced with phenobarbital:** UBC Library Open Collections, "History of Nursing in Pacific Canada." *The Vancouver Medical Association Bulletin* (November 1952), 25.
15. **"a very rare medical condition":** Bridget Christie (Guilty Feminist), "Fighting for Hope with Bridget Christie." YouTube channel, October 11, 2021; https://www.youtube.com/watch?v=llrD5GZXNvo.
18. **And zero women:** The Coronary Drug Project Research Group, "The Coronary Drug Project: Design, Methods, and Baseline Results." *Circulation* 47, no. 3 suppl. (1973): I1–I50; doi: 10.1161/01.CIR.47.3S1.I-1.
18. **British historian Louise Foxcroft:** Louise Foxcroft, *Hot Flushes, Cold Science: A History of the Modern Menopause* (London: Granta UK, 2010), 15.
18. **In a now-famous episode of *Inside Amy Schumer*:** *Inside Amy Schumer*, season 3, episode 1, "Last F**kable Day," aired April 21, 2015, on Paramount+; https://www.youtube.com/watch?v=XPpsI8mWKmg.
20. **around 30 million U.S. women:** Statista Research Department, "Resident Population of the United States by Sex and Age as of July 1, 2021." Statista, July 2022; https://www.statista.com/statistics/241488/population-of-the-us-by-sex-and-age/.

20. **birth rates have been dropping:** "Why Is the U.S. Birth Rate Declining?" PRB, US Census/American Community Survey, May 6, 2021; https://www.prb.org/resources/why-is-the-u-s-birth-rate-declining/.
20. **one in six adults over fifty-five are child-free:** Tayelor Valerio, Brian Knop, Rose M. Kreider, and Wan He, "Childless Older Americans: 2018." United States Census Bureau, Report Number P70-173 (August 31, 2021); https://www.census.gov/library/publications/2021/demo/p70-173.html.
20. **average age of menopause is fifty-one:** National Institutes of Health, "About Menopause," November 16, 2021, https://www.nichd.nih.gov/health/topics/menopause/conditioninfo.
20. **average life expectancy of a woman in the United States:** Elizabeth Arias, Betzaida Tejada-Vera, and Farida Ahmad, "Vital Statistics Rapid Release: Provisional Life Expectancy Estimates for January through June, 2020," Centers for Disease Control and Prevention (CDC), Report Number 010, February 2021; https://www.cdc.gov/nchs/data/vsrr/VSRR10-508.pdf.
21. **more than a billion women around the world:** Jan L. Shifren and Margery L. S. Gass, "The North American Menopause Society Recommendations for Clinical Care of Midlife Women." *Menopause* 21, no. 10 (2014): 1038–62; doi: 10.1097/GME.0000000000000319.

CHAPTER 2: WHY DIDN'T I KNOW THIS?

22. **five pounds on average:** Office on Women's Health, "Menopause and Your Health." U.S. Department of Health and Human Services, February 22, 2021; https://www.womenshealth.gov/menopause/menopause-and-your-health.
24. **"somebody put a furnace in my core":** Allyson Chiu, "Experts Are Cheering Michelle Obama's Openness About Hot Flashes. And They Have Some Advice." *Washington Post,* August 20, 2020; https://www.washingtonpost.com/lifestyle/wellness/michelle-obama-menopause-hot-flashes/2020/08/20/736cb23c-e195-11ea-8dd2-d07812bf00f7_story.html.
25. **they experience formication:** Pragya A. Nair, "Dermatosis Associated with Menopause." *Journal of Mid-Life Health* 5, no. 4 (2014): 168–75; doi: 10.4103/0976-7800.145152.
25. **the function of a woman's vocal cords:** Anoop Raj et al., "A Study of Voice Changes in Various Phases of Menstrual Cycle and in Postmenopausal Women." *Journal of Voice* 24, no. 3 (2010): 363–68; doi: 10.1016/j.jvoice.2008.10.005.
25. **menopausal hormone therapy can reverse:** Abdul-Latif Hamdan et al., "Effect of Hormonal Replacement Therapy on Voice." *Journal of Voice* 31, no. 1 (2018): 116–21; doi: 10.1016/j.jvoice.2017.02.019.

26. **English opera singer Lesley Garrett:** Peter Robertson, "Lesley Garrett: 'HRT Made Me a Better Singer.'" *Express UK*, June 29, 2015. https://www.express.co.uk/life-style/health/587599/lesley-garrett-opera-uk-hrt-menopause-health-women-aging.
26. **pioneering Study of Women's Health Across the Nation:** Samar R. El Khoudary et al., "The Menopause Transition and Women's Health at Midlife: A Progress Report from the Study of Women's Health Across the Nation (SWAN)." *Menopause* 26, no. 10 (2019): 1213–27; doi: 10.1097/GME.0000000000001424.
26. **A 2022 SWAN study found that Black women:** Siobán D. Harlow et al., "Disparities in Reproductive Aging and Midlife Health Between Black and White Women: The Study of Women's Health Across the Nation (SWAN)." *Women's Midlife Health* 8, no. 1 (2022): 3. doi: 10.1186/s40695-022-00073-y.
26. **three times more likely to undergo premature menopause:** "Early Menopause Linked to Higher Risk of Future Coronary Heart Disease," American Heart Association, May 20, 2021; https://newsroom.heart.org/news/early-menopause-linked-to-higher-risk-of-future-coronary-heart-disease.
27. **"Upside Down":** Snoop Dogg, "Upside Down," accessed July 8, 2022; https://www.lyrics.com/lyric/31132145/Snoop+Dogg/Upside+Down.
27. **"Jack U Off":** Prince, "Jack U Off," accessed July 8, 2022; https://www.lyrics.com/lyric/2743965/Prince/Jack+U+Off.
27. ***All in the Family* broke ground:** A. Fusco, "*All in the Family*—Edith's Problem—1972," YouTube, 2021, 4:58; https://www.youtube.com/watch?v=l_ygPP_pxr0.
28. **the episode, which won an Emmy:** Donna McCrohan, *Archie & Edith, Mike & Gloria: The Tumultuous History of* All in the Family (New York: Workman Publishing, 1988), 36.
28. **writes TV critic David Mello:** David Mello, "*All in the Family*: 10 Things You Didn't Know About the Episode 'Edith's Problem.'" Screen Rant, March 17, 2020; https://screenrant.com/all-family-ediths-problem-episode-facts-trivia/.
28. **Clair Huxtable tells her children:** Minniecia Minnie Winston, "The Cosby Show: Clair's Liberation." YouTube, June 15, 2021, 2:50; https://www.youtube.com/watch?v=vcP-5erw6Uo.
28. **In a now-famous monologue from a 2019 episode of *Fleabag*:** BBC Three, "Why You Should Look Forward to the Menopause: *Fleabag* Series 2." YouTube, March 19, 2019, 1:01; https://www.youtube.com/watch?v=RZrnHnASRV8.
28. **postmenopausal zest:** Barbara Brotman and Tribune Staff Writer, "(The) Change Is Good." *Chicago Tribune*, July 21, 1999; https://www.chicagotribune.com/news/ct-xpm-1999-07-21-9907210001-story.html.
29. **In the 2021 miniseries *Nine Perfect Strangers*:** David Bianculli, "'Nine Perfect Strangers' Is the Latest Show from the 'Big Little Lies' Team." National Public

Radio, August 16, 2021; https://www.npr.org/2021/08/16/1028101133/nine-perfect-strangers-is-the-latest-show-from-the-big-little-lies-team.

29. **One exception is a 2022 episode of *Black-ish*:** *Black-ish*, season 8, episode 11, "The (Almost) Last Dance," written by Kenya Barris, Courtney Lilly, and Tracee Ellis Ross, aired April 6, 2022, on ABC, https://abc.com/shows/blackish/episode-guide/season-08/11-the-almost-last-dance.

30. **Eric Verdin, CEO of the Buck Institute:** Guy Kovnar, "Rush of Research, Investment in Human Longevity Comes to San Francisco Bay Area." *North Bay Business Journal*, December 18, 2018; https://www.northbaybusinessjournal.com/article/industry-news/rush-of-research-investment-in-human-longevity-comes-to-san-francisco-bay/.

30. **1 to 2 percent a year from about the age of forty:** Roger D. Stanworth and T. Hugh Jones, "Testosterone for the Aging Male; Current Evidence and Recommended Practice." *Clinical Interventions in Aging* 3, no. 1 (March 2008): 25–44; doi: 10.2147/cia.s190.

30. **"It is now time for a decent burial":** John B. McKinlay et al., "Male Menopause—Time for a Decent Burial?" *Menopause* 14, no. 6 (2007): 973–75; doi: 10.1097/gme.0b013e31815708ee.

30. **grandmother hypothesis:** K. Hawkes et al., "Grandmothering, Menopause, and the Evolution of Human Life Histories." *Proceedings of the National Academy of Sciences of the United States of America* 95, no. 3 (1998): 1336–39; doi: 10.1073/pnas.95.3.1336.

31. **menopause that's induced by a medical treatment:** Cristina Secosan et al., "Surgically Induced Menopause—A Practical Review of Literature." *Medicina* 55, no. 8 (2019): 482; doi: 10.3390/medicina55080482.

32. **as early as thirty-five:** "Perimenopause." Centre for Menstrual Cycle and Ovulation Research, accessed July 8, 2022; https://www.cemcor.ca/resources/life-phases/perimenopause.

32. **participants tended to "increase their alcohol consumption":** Matti Hyvärinen et al., "Predicting the Age at Natural Menopause in Middle-Aged Women." *Menopause* 28, no. 7 (2021): 792–99; doi: 10.1097/GME.0000000000001774.

34. **Sea creature fun facts:** University of Exeter, "Beluga Whales and Narwhals Go Through Menopause." Science Daily, August 27, 2018; https://www.sciencedaily.com/releases/2018/08/180827080847.htm.

34. **postmenopausal killer whales have the biggest impact:** Stuart Nattrass et al., "Postreproductive Killer Whale Grandmothers Improve the Survival of Their Grandoffspring." *Proceedings of the National Academy of Sciences of the United States of America* 116, no. 52 (2019): 26669–73; doi: 10.1073/pnas.1903844116.

35. **"far too early for me":** Nicki Gostin, "Naomi Watts 'Wasn't Prepared' When

Menopause Hit 'Far Too Early.'" *Page Six*, June 11, 2022; https://pagesix.com/2022/06/11/naomi-watts-wasnt-prepared-when-menopause-hit-far-too-early/.

37. **your risk for conditions such as high blood pressure:** Kathy Katella, "Heart Disease in Women: How Pregnancy, Menopause, and Other Factors Affect Risk." Yale Medicine, March 3, 2022; https://www.yalemedicine.org/news/heart-disease-women.
37. **and osteoporosis rises:** "Osteoporosis: What You Need to Know as You Age." Johns Hopkins Medicine, accessed July 8, 2022; https://www.hopkinsmedicine.org/health/conditions-and-diseases/osteoporosis/osteoporosis-what-you-need-to-know-as-you-age.

CHAPTER 3: THE TWILIGHT SAGA

42. **Some six thousand women a day:** Rene Wisley, "Dealing with Perimenopause? 7 Things to Know." Michigan Health, October 25, 2021; https://healthblog.uofmhealth.org/womens-health/dealing-perimenopause-7-things-to-know.
42. **A 2022 survey from Bonafide:** "The State of Menopause." Bonafide, 2022, https://hellobonafide.com/pages/state-of-menopause-2022.
42. **The word didn't appear in *The New York Times* until 1997:** Alix Boyle, "Making a Case for Estrogen Replacement." *New York Times*, June 8, 1997; https://www.nytimes.com/1997/06/08/nyregion/making-a-case-for-estrogen-replacement.html.
42. **just 29.7 percent of Microsoft's global workforce:** Lindsay-Rae McIntyre, "Microsoft's Diversity & Inclusion Report: Demonstrating Progress and Remaining Accountable to Our Commitments." Microsoft, last modified October 20, 2021; https://blogs.microsoft.com/blog/2021/10/20/microsofts-2021-diversity-inclusion-report-demonstrating-progress-and-remaining-accountable-to-our-commitments.
43. **Alexa will now give an answer to the question:** "*Menopause Matters* Information Now Available via Amazon Alexa." Menopause Matters, May 2022; https://www.menopausematters.co.uk/pdf/alexa10May2022.pdf.
43. **perimenopause is an "ill-defined time period":** Nanette Santoro, "Perimenopause: From Research to Practice." *Journal of Women's Health* 25, no. 4 (2016): 332–39; doi: 10.1089/jwh.2015.5556.
43. **women's salaries are highest at age forty-four:** Teresa Perez, "Earnings Peak at Different Ages for Different Demographic Groups." PayScale, June 4, 2019, https://www.payscale.com/research-and-insights/peak-earnings/.

43. **defined by the Johns Hopkins website:** "Periomenopause." Johns Hopkins Medicine, accessed July 8, 2022; https://www.hopkinsmedicine.org/health/conditions-and-diseases/perimenopause.
44. **"the hormonal changes happening, the sweating, the moods":** goop, "Meet Madame Ovary." Facebook, October 29, 2018, 1:01. https://m.facebook.com/watch/?v=728165190883577&_rdr.
45. **dramatic uptick in bleeding:** Lara Delamater and Nanette Santoro, "Management of the Periomenopause." *Clinical Obstetrics and Gynecology* 61, no. 3 (2018): 419–32; doi: 10.1097/GRF.0000000000000389.
45. **prolonged bleeding for ten or more days:** Laurel Thomas, "Prolonged and Heavy Bleeding During Menopause Is Common." University of Michigan, April 15, 2014; https://news.umich.edu/prolonged-and-heavy-bleeding-during-menopause-is-common/.
45. **"No Strings Attached":** Glenn Garner and Julie Mazziotta, "'AJLT' Writers on the Real-Life Experience That Inspired Charlotte's 'Flash Period'—And What to Know." February 1, 2022; https://people.com/health/and-just-like-that-writers-real-life-experience-inspired-charlotte-flash-period/.
46. **similar to when their mothers did:** Harold Bae, "Genetic Associations with Age of Menopause in Familial Longevity," *Menopause* 26, no. 10 (2019); https://journals.lww.com/menopausejournal/toc/2019/10000.
46. **no indication that use of oral contraceptives:** E. de Vries et al., "Oral Contraceptive Use in Relation to Age at Menopause in the DOM Cohort." *Human Reproduction* 16, no. 8 (2001): 1657–62; doi: 10.1093/humrep/16.8.1657.
46. **hide or control some of the symptoms of menopause:** "How Do I Know I've Reached Menopause If I'm on the Pill?" UK National Health Service, July 1, 2020; https://www.nhs.uk/conditions/contraception/menopause-contraceptive-pill/.
46. **usually not helpful:** North American Menopause Society, *The Menopause Guidebook,* 9th ed. (Pepper Pike, OH, 2020), 3.
46. **ovaries produce estrogen:** North American Menopause Society, *The Menopause Guidebook,* 9th ed., 11.
47. **you can absolutely still get pregnant:** "Periomenopause." Cleveland Clinic, October 5, 2021; https://my.clevelandclinic.org/health/diseases/21608-perimenopause.
47. **researchers at Monash University in Clayton, Australia:** N. Bellofiore et al., "First Evidence of a Menstruating Rodent: The Spiny Mouse (*Acomys cahirinus*)." *American Journal of Obstetrics & Gynecology* 216, no. 1 (2017): 40.E1–40.E11; doi: 10.1016/j.ajog.2016.07.041.
48. **spiny mice have a gradual:** Nadia Bellofiore et al., "Reproductive Aging and Menopause-like Transition in the Menstruating Spiny Mouse (*Acomys cahirinus*)." *Human Reproduction* 36, no. 12 (2021): 3083–94; doi: 10.1093/humrep/deab215.

48. **Iron-deficiency anemia is common:** Tatnai Burnett, "Heavy Periods: Can Folic Acid Help?" Mayo Clinic, September 8, 2021; https://www.mayoclinic.org/diseases-conditions/menorrhagia/expert-answers/heavy-periods/faq-20058365.
48. **One is tranexamic acid (Lysteda):** "Tranexamic Acid (Oral Route)." Mayo Clinic, February 1, 2022; https://www.mayoclinic.org/drugs-supplements/tranexamic-acid-oral-route/proper-use/drg-20073517?p=1.
48. **reduce bleeding by about half:** Henri Leminen and Ritva Hurskainen, "Tranexamic Acid for the Treatment of Heavy Menstrual Bleeding: Efficacy and Safety." *International Journal of Women's Health* 4 (2012): 413–21; doi: 10.2147/IJWH.S13840.
48. **ibuprofen, surprisingly, has been shown to decrease:** "Quick Dose: Can Ibuprofen Reduce Menstrual Flow?" Northwestern Medicine, February 2020; https://www.nm.org/healthbeat/healthy-tips/can-ibuprofen-reduce-menstrual-flow.
49. **it doesn't have to be replaced for three to seven years:** "What Are Hormonal IUDs?" Planned Parenthood, accessed July 8, 2022; https://www.plannedparenthood.org/learn/birth-control/iud/hormonal-iuds.
49. **Tracey Thorn sings:** Tracey Thorn, "Hormones." Lyrics.com, 2015; https://www.lyrics.com/lyric/32286697/Tracey+Thorn/Hormones.
49. **first-time mother:** https://www.pewresearch.org/fact-tank/2018/06/28/u-s-women-are-postponing-motherhood-but-not-as-much-as-those-in-most-other-developed-nations.
50. **As financier Bernard M. Baruch aptly put it:** Bernard M. Baruch, "Thoughts on the Business of Life." *Forbes* Quotes, accessed July 18, 2022; https://www.forbes.com/quotes/1159/.
51. **"the rites of passage that they are":** Julie Mazziotta, "Gillian Anderson on Dealing with Early Menopause: 'I Felt Like Somebody Else Had Taken over My Brain.'" *People*, March 13, 2017; https://people.com/health/gillian-anderson-perimenopause-depression/.
52. **this fuzziness tends to clear up:** Eva Schelbaum et al., "Association of Reproductive History with Brain MRI Biomarkers of Dementia Risk in Midlife." *Neurology* 97, no. 23 (2021): e2328–e2339; doi: 10.1212/WNL.0000000000012941.
52. **"Emotional sensitivity to psychosocial stress":** Jennifer L. Gordon et al., "Estradiol Variability, Stressful Life Events, and the Emergence of Depressive Symptomatology During the Menopausal Transition." *Menopause* 23, no. 3 (2016): 257–66; doi: 10.1097/GME.0000000000000528.
52. **they're nearly twice as likely:** Mayo Clinic Staff, "Depression in Women: Understanding the Gender Gap." Mayo Clinic, January 29, 2019; https://www.mayoclinic.org/diseases-conditions/depression/in-depth/depression/art-20047725.

52. **A 2021 study in the journal *Psychoneuroendocrinology*:** Anouk E. de Wit et al., "Predictors of Irritability Symptoms in Mildly Depressed Perimenopausal Women." *Psychoneuroendocrinology* 126 (2021): 105128; doi: 10.1016/j.psyneuen.2021.105128.
52. **twice as likely to show up when perimenopause begins:** Lee S. Cohen et al., "Risk for New Onset of Depression During the Menopausal Transition." *Archives of General Psychiatry* 63, no. 4 (2006): 385–90; doi: 10.1001/archpsyc.63.4.385.
53. **clinical guidelines were finally published in 2018:** Sharon Parmet, "First-Ever Guidelines for Detecting, Treating Perimenopausal Depression." UIC Today, September 5, 2018; https://today.uic.edu/first-ever-guidelines-for-detecting-treating-perimenopausal-depression.
53. **The average doctor's visit lasts eighteen minutes:** Hannah T. Neprash et al., "Measuring Primary Care Exam Length Using Electronic Health Record Data." *Medical Care* 59, no. 1 (2021): 62–66; doi: 10.1097/MLR.0000000000001450.
54. **Over-the-counter tests usually measure follicle-stimulating hormone (FSH):** North American Menopause Society, *The Menopause Guidebook*, 9th ed., 3.
54. **NAMS's position on its website is pretty straightforward:** "What Is Hormone Testing?" North American Menopause Society, accessed July 8, 2022; https://www.menopause.org/publications/clinical-practice-materials/bioidentical-hormone-therapy/what-is-hormone-testing-.
54. **A helpful way to figure out:** Christie Aschwanden, "Hormone Therapy, Long Shunned for a Possible Breast Cancer Link, Is Now Seen as a Short-Term Treatment for Menopause Symptoms." *Washington Post*, February 29, 2020, https://www.washingtonpost.com/health/hormone-therapy-long-shunned-for-a-possible-breast-cancer-link-is-now-seen-as-safe-and-helpful-as-a-short-term-treatment-for-most-women-in-the-throes-of-menopause/2020/02/28/1fd19f66-54cd-11ea-929a-64efa7482a77_story.html.
55. **more likely to be prescribed hormone therapy:** Anna Blanken et al., "Racial/Ethnic Disparities in the Diagnosis and Management of Menopause Symptoms Among Midlife Women Veterans." *Menopause* 29, no. 7 (2022): 877–82; doi: 10.1097/GME.0000000000001978.
55. **A Penn Medicine analysis:** Lauren Ingeno, "Study Finds Patients Prefer Doctors Who Share Their Same Race/Ethnicity." Penn Medicine News, November 9, 2020; https://www.pennmedicine.org/news/news-releases/2020/november/study-finds-patients-prefer-doctors-who-share-their-same-race-ethnicity.
57. **Some symptoms of hyperthyroidism:** "Is It Menopause or a Thyroid Problem?" North American Menopause Society, accessed July 8, 2022, https://www.menopause.org/for-women/menopauseflashes/menopause-symptoms-and-treatments/is-it-menopause-or-a-thyroid-problem.

57. **If you have a history of osteoporosis:** Rachel Nall, "Does Medicare Cover Bone Density Tests?" Medical News Today, October 21, 2020; https://www.medicalnewstoday.com/articles/does-medicare-cover-bone-density-test.
58. **the FDA-approved Brisdelle:** Ronald J. Orleans et al., "FDA Approval of Paroxetine for Menopausal Hot Flushes." *New England Journal of Medicine* 370 (2014): 1777–79; doi: 10.1056/NEJMp1402080.
58. **a 2020 meta-analysis of the antiseizure medication gabapentin:** Sang-Hee Yoon et al., "Gabapentin for the Treatment of Hot Flushes in Menopause: A Meta-Analysis." *Menopause* 27, no. 4 (April 2020): 485–93; doi: 10.1097/GME.0000000000001491.
58. **For vaginal dryness:** North American Menopause Society, *The Menopause Guidebook,* 9th ed., 35.
58. **researchers at the University of Copenhagen:** Department of Nutrition, Exercise, and Sports, "Blood Vessel Growth in Muscle Is Reduced in Women After Menopause." University of Copenhagen, September 22, 2020; https://nexs.ku.dk/english/news/2020/blood-vessel-growth-in-muscle-is-reduced-in-women-after-menopause/.
58. **the greatest increases:** Lacey M. Gould et al., "Metabolic Effects of Menopause: A Cross-Sectional Characterization of Body Composition and Exercise Metabolism." *Menopause* 29, no. 4 (2022): 377–89; doi: 10.1097/GME.0000000000001932.
59. **"comparable with pharmacological interventions":** Luigi Barrea et al., "Mediterranean Diet as Medical Prescription in Menopausal Women with Obesity: A Practical Guide for Nutritionists." *Critical Reviews in Food Science and Nutrition* 61, no. 7 (2020): 1201–11; doi: 10.1080/10408398.2020.1755220.
59. **tracked more than 14,000 British women:** Yashvee Dunneram et al., "Dietary Intake and Age at Natural Menopause: Results from the UK Women's Cohort Study." *Journal of Epidemiology and Community Health* 72, no. 8 (2018): 733–40; doi: 10.1136/jech-2017-209887.
59. **up to 20 percent of their bone density:** "Menopause and Bone Loss." Endocrine Society, January 24, 2022; https://www.endocrine.org/patient-engagement/endocrine-library/menopause-and-bone-loss.
59. **1,200 milligrams of calcium a day:** "Calcium and Vitamin D: Important at Every Age." NIH Osteoporosis and Related Bone Diseases National Resource Center, October 2018, https://www.bones.nih.gov/health-info/bone/bone-health/nutrition/calcium-and-vitamin-d-important-every-age.
59. **Greek yogurt may have a better reputation:** The Nutrition Source, "Yogurt." Harvard T. H. Chan School of Public Health, accessed July 8, 2022; https://www.hsph.harvard.edu/nutritionsource/food-features/yogurt/.
59. **recommend 600 IU of vitamin D:** National Institutes of Health, Office of Di-

etary Supplements, "Vitamin D." Last updated August 12, 2022; https://ods.od.nih.gov/factsheets/VitaminD-HealthProfessional/.

59. **one in *two* women:** Bone Health & Osteoporosis Foundation, "What Women Need to Know." Accessed July 8, 2022; https://www.bonehealthandosteoporosis.org/preventing-fractures/general-facts/what-women-need-to-know.
60. **defined by the U.S. Dietary Guidelines as one drink a day:** "Dietary Guidelines for Alcohol." Center for Disease Control and Prevention, April 19, 2022, https://www.cdc.gov/alcohol/fact-sheets/moderate-drinking.htm.
60. **a 2020 SWAN study of alcohol use among women:** MacKenzie R. Peltier, "Changes in Excessive Alcohol Use Among Older Women Across the Menopausal Transition: A Longitudinal Analysis of the Study of Women's Health Across the Nation." *Biology of Sex Differences* 11, no. 1 (2020): 37; doi: 10.1186/s13293-020-00314-7.
60. **Smoking has been shown, in a study of 79,000 women:** "Smoking 'Linked to Earlier Menopause.'" BBC News, December 16, 2015; https://www.bbc.com/news/health-35102117.
60. **Women who have sex weekly:** Natasha Downes, "Having Less Sex Linked to Earlier Menopause." University College London News, January 15, 2020; https://www.ucl.ac.uk/news/2020/jan/having-less-sex-linked-earlier-menopause.
61. **Cher, who once tweeted that:** Cher (@cher), "Ok..being older than METHUSELAH." Twitter, May 21, 2015; https://twitter.com/cher/status/601375635781459968?lang=en.

CHAPTER 4: YOUR SMOKIN' HOT NEW BODY

68. **plague up to 80 percent**: Ramandeep Bansal and Neelam Aggarwal, "Menopausal Hot Flashes: A Concise Review." *Journal of Mid-Life Health* 10, no. 1 (2019): 6–13; doi: 10.4103/jmh.JMH_7_19.
68. **lasts between one and five minutes:** Mayo Clinic Staff, "Hot Flashes." Mayo Clinic, May 20, 2022; https://www.mayoclinic.org/diseases-conditions/hot-flashes/symptoms-causes/syc-20352790.
68. **"*a small proportion of women will never be free of them*":** Nanette Santoro, "Perimenopause: From Research to Practice." *Journal of Women's Health* 25, no. 4 (2016): 332–39; doi: 10.1089/jwh.2015.5556.
68. **when plunging estrogen levels:** Mayo Clinic Staff, "Hot Flashes."
69. **"The hot flashes are the worst":** Wanda Sykes, "Wanda Sykes: Not Normal (2019)—Full Transcript." Scraps from the Loft, May 22, 2019; https://scrapsfromtheloft.com/comedy/wanda-sykes-not-normal-transcript/.

70. **tactile hallucinations:** Dani Blum, "How to Recognize and Treat Perimenopause and Menopause Symptoms." *New York Times*, April 29, 2021; https://www.nytimes.com/2021/04/29/well/perimenopause-menopause-symptoms.html.
70. **women can be blasted:** Marie Suszynski, "Menopause and Sweating." Web MD, July 20, 2011; https://www.webmd.com/menopause/features/menopause-sweating-11.
71. **persisting into their sixties, seventies, and eighties:** Jim McVeigh, "News Flash about Hot Flashes: They Can Last Longer Than You Think." Mayo Clinic, May 31, 2018; https://newsnetwork.mayoclinic.org/discussion/news-flash-about-hot-flashes-they-can-last-longer-than-you-think/.
71. **women of Chinese and Japanese descent:** Nancy E. Avis et al., "Duration of Menopausal Vasomotor Symptoms Over the Menopause Transition." *JAMA Internal Medicine* 175, no. 4 (2015): 531–39; doi: 10.1001/jamainternmed.2014.8063.
71. **a quarter century of research:** Siobán D. Harlow et al., "Disparities in Reproductive Aging and Midlife Health Between Black and White Women: The Study of Women's Health Across the Nation (SWAN)." *Women's Midlife Health* 8, no. 1 (2022): 3; doi: 10.1186/s40695-022-00073-y.
72. **women who experience frequent or persistent hot flashes:** Rebecca C. Thurston et al., "Menopausal Vasomotor Symptoms and Risk of Incident Cardiovascular Disease Events in SWAN." *Journal of the American Heart Association* 10, no. 3 (2021): e017416; doi: 10.1161/JAHA.120.017416.
72. **it's not breast cancer:** "Survey: Many Don't Realize Heart Disease Is #1 Killer for Women (PKG)." Cleveland Clinic Newsroom, January 31, 2020; https://newsroom.clevelandclinic.org/2020/01/31/survey-many-dont-realize-heart-disease-is-1-killer-for-women-pkg.
73. **Progesterone reduces the risk of uterine cancer:** North American Menopause Society, *The Menopause Guidebook,* 9th ed. (Pepper Pike, OH, 2020), 25.
73. **menopausal hormone therapy prescribed before the age of sixty:** Mayo Clinic Staff, "Hormone Therapy: Is It Right for You?" Mayo Clinic, June 3, 2022; https://www.mayoclinic.org/diseases-conditions/menopause/in-depth/hormone-therapy/art-20046372.
74. **such as weight gain:** David J. Portman et al., "Effects of Low-Dose Paroxetine 7.5 mg on Weight and Sexual Function During Treatment of Vasomotor Symptoms Associated with Menopause." *Menopause* 21, no. 10 (2014): 1082–90; doi: 10.1097/GME.0000000000000210.
74. **The term *off-label:*** "Off-Label Drugs: What You Need to Know." Agency for Healthcare Research and Quality, September 2015; https://www.ahrq.gov/patients-consumers/patient-involvement/off-label-drug-usage.html.

75. **In the study that Dhillo led:** Manish Modi and Waljit S. Dhillo, "Neurokinin B and Neurokinin-3 Receptor Signaling: Promising Developments in the Management of Menopausal Hot Flushes." *Seminars in Reproductive Medicine* 37, no. 3 (2019): 125–30; doi: 10.1055/s-0039-3400241.

75. **a mind-blowing three days:** Imperial Biomedical Research Centre, "New Class of Menopause Drugs Reduces Number and Severity of Hot Flushes in Just Three Days." National Institute for Health and Care Research, March 19, 2018; https://imperialbrc.nihr.ac.uk/2018/03/19/new-class-of-menopause-drugs-reduces-number-and-severity-of-hot-flushes-in-just-three-days/.

75. **A 2020 study led by Dr. Santoro:** Nanette Santoro et al., "Effect of the Neurokinin 3 Receptor Antagonist Fezolinetant on Patient-Reported Outcomes in Postmenopausal Women with Vasomotor Symptoms: Results of a Randomized, Placebo-Controlled, Double-Blind, Dose-Ranging Study (VESTA)." *Menopause* 27, no. 12 (2020): 1350–56; doi: 10.1097/GME.0000000000001621.

79. **NAMS lists a number:** Terry M. Gibbs, "Breast Cancer Survivors & Hot Flash Treatments." North American Menopause Society, July 8, 2022; https://www.menopause.org/for-women/menopauseflashes/menopause-symptoms-and-treatments/breast-cancer-survivors-hot-flash-treatments.

79. **stellate ganglion block may be worth investigating:** North American Menopause Society, *The Menopause Guidebook,* 9th ed., 24.

80. **"My mom is eighty-three":** Craig McLean, "Interview: Stevie Nicks: The Men, the Music, the Menopause." *The Guardian*, March 25, 2011, https://www.theguardian.com/music/2011/mar/25/stevie-nicks-interview.

82. **reducing the frequency and severity of hot flashes:** Belinda H. Jenks et al., "A Pilot Study on the Effects of *S*-Equol Compared to Soy Isoflavones on Menopausal Hot Flash Frequency." *Journal of Women's Health* 21, no. 6 (2012): 674–82; doi: 10.1089/jwh.2011.3153.

82. **you must wait two to three months:** "Clinical Research." Equelle, July 8, 2022; https://equelle.com/pages/clinical-research.

82. **what *Consumer Reports* experts say:** Kevin Loria, "How to Choose Supplements Wisely." *Consumer Reports*, October 30, 2019; https://www.consumerreports.org/supplements/how-to-choose-supplements-wisely-a2238386100/.

82. **27 percent were using cannabis:** Brian P. Dunleavy, "Survey: 1 in 4 Women Use Cannabis to Manage Menopause Symptoms." United Press International, September 28, 2020; https://www.upi.com/Health_News/2020/09/28/Survey-1-in-4-women-use-cannabis-to-manage-menopause-symptoms/4271601298812/.

83. **a Schedule 1 drug:** "Drug Fact Sheet: Marijuana/Cannabis." Department of Justice/Drug Enforcement Administration, April 2020, 3; https://www.dea.gov/sites/default/files/2020-06/Marijuana-Cannabis-2020_0.pdf.

83. **In a 2021 review:** Javier Mejia-Gomez et al., "Effect of Cannabis Use in Peri- and Post-Menopausal Women: A Systematic Review," *Journal of Obstetrics and Gynaecology Canada* 43, no. 5 (2021), 680-81; doi: 10.1016/j.jogc.2021.02.107.
84. **"know that it's not risk-free"**: Lauren Streicher, *Hot Flash Hell* (Independently published, August 31, 2021), 95.
84. **The most common, according to the Cleveland Clinic:** "Hot Flashes." Cleveland Clinic, March 21, 2022; https://my.clevelandclinic.org/health/articles/15223-hot-flashes.
84. **Research presented at the NAMS annual conference in 2021:** Linnea Duley, "Prof. Sarah Witkowski: Alleviating Symptoms of Menopause." Grécourt Gate, October 29, 2021; https://www.smith.edu/news/prof-sarah-witkowski-alleviating-symptoms-menopause.
85. **But when women do manage to quit, studies show:** Rebecca L. Smith, Jodi A. Flaws, and Lisa Gallicchio, "Does Quitting Smoking Decrease the Risk of Midlife Hot Flashes? A Longitudinal Analysis." *Maturitas* 82, no. 1 (2015): 123–27; doi: 10.1016/j.maturitas.2015.06.029.
85. **Paced breathing:** Debra S. Burns and Janet S. Carpenter, "Paced Respiration for Hot Flashes?" *The Female Patient* 37 (July/August 2012): 38–41; https://www.menopause.org/docs/professional/tfppaced0712.pdf.
85. **diaphragmatic breathing:** Xiao Ma et al., "The Effect of Diaphragmatic Breathing on Attention, Negative Affect and Stress in Healthy Adults." *Frontiers in Psychology* 8 (2017): 874; doi: 10.3389/fpsyg.2017.00874.
86. **positive self-talk:** Esmaeil Sadri Damirchi et al., "The Role of Self-Talk in Predicting Death Anxiety, Obsessive-Compulsive Disorder, and Coping Strategies in the Face of Coronavirus Disease (COVID-19)." *Iranian Journal of Psychiatry* 15, no. 3 (2020): 182–88; doi: 10.18502/ijps.v15i3.3810.
87. **participants used *you* or their own names:** Jason S. Moser et al., "Third-Person Self-Talk Facilitates Emotion Regulation Without Engaging Cognitive Control: Converging Evidence from ERP and fMRI." *Scientific Reports* 7 (2017): 4519; doi: 10.1038/s41598-017-04047-3.

CHAPTER 5: I DIDN'T GET ANY SLEEP, BUT I DID CATCH UP ON MY BROODING

91. **"Did I have night sweats?":** Marlo Thomas, "Dealing with Menopause, from Rosie O'Donnell." YouTube, 1:59; https://www.youtube.com/watch?v=uSk8xg-Tz0I.
92. **considerably more common in women:** Bin Zhang and Yun-Kwok Wing, "Sex Differences in Insomnia: A Meta-Analysis." *Sleep* 29, no. 1 (2006): 85–93; doi: 10.1093/sleep/29.1.85.

92. **a 2018 study:** Snigdha Pusalavidyasagar et al., "Sleep in Women Across the Stages of Life." *Clinical Pulmonary Medicine* 25, no. 3 (2018): 89–99; doi 10.1097/CPM.0000000000000263.
92. **Matthew Walker, author of *Why We Sleep*:** "'Catastrophic' Lack of Sleep in Modern Society Is Killing Us, Warns Leading Sleep Scientist." Association of Flight Attendants, September 25, 2017; https://www.afacwa.org/lack_of_sleep_killing_us_warns_leading_sleep_scientist-2017.
93. **the risks of developing heart disease, stroke, high blood pressure, and type 2 diabetes:** "Sleep and Sleep Disorders." Centers for Disease Control and Prevention, September 7, 2022; https://www.cdc.gov/sleep/index.html.
93. **menopause o'clock:** Samantha Irby (@bitchesgottaeat), "deliriously awake at menopause o'clock," January 20, 2021; https://www.instagram.com/p/CKQd0Kgg2Zf/?hl=en.
94. **first-year medical residents:** Yu Fang et al., "Day-to-Day Variability in Sleep Parameters and Depression Risk: A Prospective Cohort Study of Training Physicians." *npj Digital Medicine* 4, no. 1 (2021): 28; doi: 10.1038/s41746-021-00400-z.
95. **the decibel levels of snorers:** Mudiaga Sowho et al., "Snoring: A Source of Noise Pollution and Sleep Apnea Predictor." *Sleep* 43, no. 6 (2020): zsz305; doi: 10.1093/sleep/zsz305.
95. **sleep when their partner is nearby:** "More Couples Opting to Sleep in Separate Beds, Study Suggests." CBC, August 6, 2013; https://www.cbc.ca/news/health/more-couples-opting-to-sleep-in-separate-beds-study-suggests-1.1316019.
95. **nearly one in four:** Scott Muska, "Can Sleeping in Separate Beds Actually Be Good for Your Relationship?" Better by Today, October 9, 2017; https://www.nbcnews.com/better/health/can-sleeping-separate-beds-actually-be-good-your-relationship-ncna807261.
96. **an increasing demand:** Toll Brothers, "The Dual Primary Bedroom Trend & Why It's So Popular in Luxury Homes." Toll Brothers, August 24, 2022; https://www.tollbrothers.com/blog/dual-primary-bedrooms-a-growing-trend/.
96. **in the words of renowned sex therapist Esther Perel:** Esther Perel and Mary Alice Miller, "Feeling Alone in a Relationship? You're Not Alone." Esther Perel, accessed July 9, 2022; https://www.estherperel.com/blog/feeling-alone-in-a-relationship-youre-not-alone.
97. **used by an estimated one-fifth of Americans with chronic insomnia:** Timothy Roehrs and Thomas Roth, "Insomnia as a Path to Alcoholism: Tolerance Development and Dose Escalation." *Sleep* 41, no. 8 (2018); doi: 10.1093/sleep/zsy091.
97. **people who drink before bed often experience:** Ian M. Colrain, Christian L. Nicholas, and Fiona C. Baker, "Alcohol and the Sleeping Brain." *Handbook of Clinical Neurology* 125 (2014): 415–31; doi: 10.1016/B978-0-444-62619-6.00024-0.

97. **four hours before heading off to bed:** "Caffeine, Food, Alcohol, Smoking and Sleep." Sleep Health Foundation, 2013; https://www.sleephealthfoundation.org.au/pdfs/CaffeineAlcohol-0713.pdf.

97. **Americans using melatonin has quadrupled:** Jingen Li et al., "Trends in Use of Melatonin Supplements Among US Adults, 1999–2018." *JAMA* 327, no. 5 (2022): 483–85; doi:10.1001/jama.2021.23652.

97. **available by prescription:** "Melatonin for Sleep Problems." National Health Service, November 8, 2019; https://www.nhs.uk/medicines/melatonin/.

98. **a mere .3 milligram:** Deborah Halber, "Scientists Pinpoint Dosage of Melatonin for Insomnia." MIT News, October 17, 2001; https://news.mit.edu/2001/melatonin-1017.

98. **according to a 2018 Australian study:** Tracey L. Sletten et al., "Efficacy of Melatonin with Behavioural Sleep-Wake Scheduling for Delayed Sleep-Wake Phase Disorder: A Double-Blind, Randomised Clinical Trial." *PLoS Medicine* 15, no. 6 (2018): e1002587; doi: 10.1371/journal.pmed.1002587.

98. **About a third of 1,500 women surveyed:** Colleen Hall, "Common Problems Associated with Menopause Alleviated with Cannabis Use, Patients Report." *Contemporary OB/GYN* 66, no. 11 (2021); https://www.contemporaryobgyn.net/view/common-problems-associated-with-menopause-alleviated-with-cannabis-use-patients-report.

98. **This, according to *Consumer Reports*, is true:** Lisa L. Gill, "Is It Safe to Vape CBD?" *Consumer Reports*, January 31, 2020; https://www.consumerreports.org/cbd/is-it-safe-to-vape-cbd/.

98. **magnesium's soporific effects:** Jasmine Mah and Tyler Pitre, "Oral Magnesium Supplementation for Insomnia in Older Adults: A Systematic Review and Meta-Analysis." *BMC Complementary Medicine and Therapies* 21, no. 1 (2021): 125; doi: 10.1186/s12906-021-03297-z.

99. **"I will wake up just soaking":** Glennon Doyle, "Menopause: What We Deserve to Know with Dr. Jen Gunter." Momastery, April 26, 2022; https://momastery.com/blog/we-can-do-hard-things-ep-90.

100. **200 milligrams of magnesium glycinate:** "Does Magnesium Help You Sleep?" Cleveland Clinic, June 29, 2021; https://health.clevelandclinic.org/does-magnesium-help-you-sleep/.

100. **A 2017 review in the journal *Sleep Science*:** Shazia Jehan et al., "Sleep, Melatonin, and the Menopausal Transition: What Are the Links?" *Sleep Science* 10, no. 1 (2017): 11–18; doi: 10.5935/1984-0063.20170003.

100. **Stanford University neuroscientist Dr. Andrew Huberman:** "The Tim Ferriss Show Transcripts: Dr. Andrew Huberman—A Neurobiologist on Optimizing Sleep, Performance, and Testosterone (#521)." *The Tim Ferriss Show*, July 8, 2021; https://tim.blog/2021/07/08/andrew-huberman-transcript/.

101. **One of the best ways to bring on sleep:** Mayo Clinic Staff, "Insomnia Treatment: Cognitive Behavioral Therapy Instead of Sleeping Pills." Mayo Clinic, September 28, 2016; https://www.mayoclinic.org/diseases-conditions/insomnia/in-depth/insomnia-treatment/art-20046677.
102. **"the bear is always there":** Ravinder Jerath, Connor Beveridge, and Vernon A. Barnes, "Self-Regulation of Breathing as an Adjunctive Treatment of Insomnia." *Frontiers in Psychiatry* 9 (January 2019): 780; doi: 10.3389/fpsyt.2018.00780.
102. **alone with your thoughts:** Rafael Pelayo, "7 Tips to Sleeping Well." TEDx-MarinSalon, YouTube, May 6, 2021, 11:51; https://www.youtube.com/watch?v=R8CNKE8nHfQ.
103. **cause a "high level of cognitive activation":** Michael K. Scullin et al., "The Effects of Bedtime Writing on Difficulty Falling Asleep: A Polysomnographic Study Comparing To-Do Lists and Completed Activity Lists." *Journal of Experimental Psychology: General* 147, no. 1 (2018): 139–46; doi: 10.1037/xge0000374.
103. **people who spent five minutes:** Scullin et al. "The Effects of Bedtime Writing on Difficulty Falling Asleep: A Polysomnographic Study Comparing To-Do Lists and Completed Activity Lists."

CHAPTER 6: 50, SHADES OF GRAY

106. **a *New York Times* article appeared:** Melinda Wenner Moyer, "Why Do Women Sprout Chin Hairs as They Age?" *New York Times*, Ask Well, December 14, 2021; https://www.nytimes.com/2021/12/14/well/live/chin-hairs-women.html.
107. **A prescription cream called Vaniqa:** "Vaniqa (Eflornithine Hydrochloride) Cream, 13.9%." Bristol-Myers Squibb Labeling, July 27, 2000; https://www.accessdata.fda.gov/drugsatfda_docs/label/2000/21145lbl.pdf.
109. **Thai researchers:** Sukanya Chaikittisilpa et al., "Prevalence of Female Pattern Hair Loss in Postmenopausal Women: A Cross-Sectional Study." *Menopause* 29, no. 4 (2022): 415–20; doi: 10.1097/GME.0000000000001927.
110. **can restore hair growth:** "Thinning Hair and Hair Loss: Could It Be Female Pattern Hair Loss?" American Academy of Dermatology Association, October 3, 2022; https://www.aad.org/public/diseases/hair-loss/types/female-pattern.
111. **"Menopause is hell, Jimmy":** "Viola Davis Explains Menopause to Jimmy Kimmel." *Jimmy Kimmel Live,* YouTube, January 30, 2019, 6:05; https://www.youtube.com/watch?v=7Uipsro4x4w.
112. **pair PRP with minoxidil:** Alison J. Bruce et al., "A Randomized, Controlled Pilot Trial Comparing Platelet-Rich Plasma to Topical Minoxidil Foam for Treatment of Androgenic Alopecia in Women." *Dermatologic Surgery* 46, no. 6 (2020): 826–32: doi: 10.1097/DSS.0000000000002168.

112. **A 2019 study:** Robert S. English Jr., and James M. Barazesh, "Self-Assessments of Standardized Scalp Massages for Androgenic Alopecia: Survey Results." *Dermatology and Therapy* 9 (2019): 167–78; doi: 10.1007/s13555-019-0281-6.
112. **thirteen studies in the *American Journal of Lifestyle Medicine*:** Roman Pawlak, Julia Berger, and Ian Hines, "Iron Status of Vegetarian Adults: A Review of Literature." *American Journal of Lifestyle Medicine* 12, no. 6 (2016): 486–98; doi: 10.1177/1559827616682933.
116. **It helps ward off osteoporosis, diabetes, and heart disease:** D. S. Siscovick, R. E. LaPorte, and J. M. Newman, "The Disease-Specific Benefits and Risks of Physical Activity and Exercise." *Public Health Reports* 100, no. 2 (1985): 180–88; https://pubmed.ncbi.nlm.nih.gov/3920716/.
116. **recommends 2.5 hours to 5 hours:** "Top 10 Things to Know About the Second Edition of the Physical Activity Guidelines for Americans," health.gov, August 25, 2021; https://health.gov/our-work/nutrition-physical-activity/physical-activity-guidelines/current-guidelines/top-10-things-know.
116. **lifesaving benefits of regular dog walking:** Hayley Christian et al., "Encouraging Dog Walking for Health Promotion and Disease Prevention." *American Journal of Lifestyle Medicine* 12, no. 3 (2016): 233–43; doi: 10.1177/1559827616643686.
116. **2021 report in the journal *Critical Reviews in Food Science and Nutrition*:** Luigi Barrea et al., "Mediterranean Diet as Medical Prescription in Menopausal Women with Obesity: A Practical Guide for Nutritionists." *Critical Reviews in Food Science and Nutrition* 61, no. 7 (2020): 1201–11; doi: 10.1080/10408398.2020.1755220.
117. **As ob-gyn Jen Gunter, author of *The Menopause Manifesto*:** Jen Gunter, "7 Fertility Myths That Belong in the Past." *New York Times*, April 15, 2020; https://www.nytimes.com/2020/04/15/parenting/fertility/trying-to-conceive-myths.html.
117. **your risk of developing high blood pressure:** Teresa A. Milner et al., "Estrogen Receptor β Contributes to Both Hypertension and Hypothalamic Plasticity in a Mouse Model of Peri-Menopause." *Journal of Neuroscience* 41, no. 24 (June 2021): 5190–5205; doi: 10.1523/JNEUROSCI.0164-21.2021.
117. **a 2018 Korean study:** S.-J. Kwon, Y.-C. Ha, and Y. Park, "High Dietary Sodium Intake Is Associated with Low Bone Mass in Postmenopausal Women: Korea National Health and Nutrition Examination Survey, 2008–2011." *Osteoporosis International* 28, no. 4 (January 2017): 1445–52; doi: 10.1007/s00198-017-3904-8.
118. **The American Heart Association recommends:** "Why Should I Limit Sodium?" American Heart Association, 2021; https://www.heart.org/-/media/files/health-topics/answers-by-heart/why-should-i-limit-sodium.pdf.

119. **the production of collagen:** Susan Stevenson and Julie Thornton, "Effect of Estrogens on Skin Aging and the Potential Role of SERMs." *Clinical Interventions in Aging* 2, no. 3 (2007): 283–97; doi: 10.2147/cia.s798.
119. **30 percent of dermal collagen:** Alexander K. Rzepecki et al., "Estrogen-Deficient Skin: The Role of Topical Therapy." *International Journal of Women's Dermatology* 5, no. 2 (2016): 85–90; doi: 10.1016/j.ijwd.2019.01.001.
119. **"Jowls appear":** "Caring for Your Skin in Menopause." American Academy of Dermatology Association, accessed July 9, 2022; https://www.aad.org/public/everyday-care/skin-care-secrets/anti-aging/skin-care-during-menopause.
120. **"Can we please do away with the 'still'?!":** Paulina Porizkova (@paulinaporizkov), "Can we please do away with the 'still'?!" Instagram, April 7, 2021; https://www.instagram.com/p/CcD24aDuVwG/.
122. **"your shape changes":** Wendy Naugle, "Andie MacDowell on Embracing Her Gray Hair: 'I Am Happier—I Really Like It.'" *People*, June 15, 2022; https://people.com/style/andie-macdowell-on-embracing-her-gray-hair-i-am-happier-i-really-like-it/.
123. **Retinol, the vitamin A derivative:** Siddharth Mukherjee et al., "Retinoids in the Treatment of Skin Aging: An Overview of Clinical Efficacy and Safety." *Clinical Interventions in Aging* 1, no. 4 (2006): 327–48; doi: 10.2147/ciia.2006.1.4.327.
124. **melanin-rich skin has lower levels:** Derrick C. Wan et al., "Moisturizing Different Racial Skin Types." *Journal of Clinical and Aesthetic Dermatology* 7, no. 6 (June 2014): 25–32; https://www.ncbi.nlm.nih.gov/pmc/articles/PMC4086530/.
125. **rich in beneficial fatty acids:** Mara Therese Padilla Evangelista, Flordeliz Abad-Casintahan, and Lillian Lopez-Villafuerte, "The Effect of Topical Virgin Coconut Oil on SCORAD Index, Transepidermal Water Loss, and Skin Capacitance in Mild to Moderate Pediatric Atopic Dermatitis: A Randomized, Double-Blind, Clinical Trial." *International Journal of Dermatology* 53, no. 1 (2014): 100–108; doi: 10.1111/ijd.12339.
126. **Peptides, which are short-chain amino acids:** Grace Gallagher, "Peptides and Your Skin Care Routine." Healthline, May 13, 2022; https://www.healthline.com/health/peptides-for-skin.
126. **a healing ingredient:** Malgorzata Litwiniuk et al., "Hyaluronic Acid in Inflammation and Tissue Regeneration." *Wounds* 28, no. 3 (2016): 78–88; https://pubmed.ncbi.nlm.nih.gov/26978861/.
127. **directly breaks down the collagen:** Ketevan Jariashvili et al., "UV Damage of Collagen: Insights from Model Collagen Peptides." *Biopolymers* 97, no. 3 (2012): 189–98; doi: 10.1002/bip.21725.

CHAPTER 7: WHY DID I WALK INTO THIS ROOM AGAIN?

130. **Nearly a quarter of women:** Eef Hogervorst, Jen Craig, and Emma O'Donnell, "Cognition and Mental Health in Menopause: A Review." *Best Practice & Research Clinical Obstetrics & Gynaecology* 81 (2021): 69–84; doi: 10.1016/j.bpobgyn.2021.10.009.
130. **Other large-scale studies:** G. A. Greendale et al., "Effects of the Menopause Transition and Hormone Use on Cognitive Performance in Midlife Women." *Neurology* 72, no. 21 (2009): 1850–57; doi: 10.1212/WNL.0b013e3181a71193.
131. **"I would get so low":** Patia Braithwaite, "Taraji P. Henson Takes on Mental Health, Menopause, and the Myth of the 'Strong Black Woman.'" *Self*, December 3, 2019; https://www.self.com/story/taraji-p-henson.
132. **Estrogen stimulates neural activity:** Bruce S. McEwen et al., "Estrogen Effects on the Brain: Actions Beyond the Hypothalamus via Novel Mechanisms." *Behavioral Neuroscience* 126, no. 1 (2012): 4–16; doi: 10.1037/a0026708.
132. **in their penises:** Chishimba N. Mowa, Subrina Jesmin, and T. Miyauchi, "The Penis: A New Target and Source of Estrogen in Male Reproduction." *Histology and Histopathology* 21, no. 1 (2006): 53–67; doi: 10.14670/HH-21.53.
133. **In a 2021 study published in the journal *Scientific Reports*:** Lisa Mosconi et al., "Menopause Impacts Human Brain Structure, Connectivity, Energy Metabolism, and Amyloid-Beta Deposition." *Scientific Reports* 11, no. 1 (2021): 10867; doi: 10.1038/s41598-021-90084-y.
135. **In his 1857 book on menopause:** Edward John Tilt, *The Change of Life in Health and Disease* (London: John Churchill and Sons, 1857), https://wellcomecollection.org/works/eyyzws59.
136. **women are already nearly twice as likely:** Mayo Clinic Staff, "Depression in Women: Understanding the Gender Gap." Mayo Clinic, January 29, 2019, https://www.mayoclinic.org/diseases-conditions/depression/in-depth/depression/art-20047725.
136. **so, too, do serotonin levels:** "Can Menopause Cause Depression?" Johns Hopkins Medicine, accessed July 9, 2022; https://www.hopkinsmedicine.org/health/wellness-and-prevention/can-menopause-cause-depression.
136. **Sandra Tsing Loh's description of menopause:** Sandra Tsing Loh, "The Bitch Is Back." *The Atlantic*, October 2011; https://www.theatlantic.com/magazine/archive/2011/10/the-bitch-is-back/308642/.
136. **if they have had a previous diagnosis:** Jennifer L. Gordon et al., "Mood Sensitivity to Estradiol Predicts Depressive Symptoms in the Menopause Transition." *Psychological Medicine* 51, no. 10 (July 2021): 1733–41; doi: 10.1017/S0033291720000483.

137. **women were two to four times:** J. T. Bromberger et al., "Major Depression During and After the Menopausal Transition: Study of Women's Health Across the Nation (SWAN)." *Psychological Medicine* 41, no. 9 (2011): 1879–88; doi: 10.1017/S003329171100016X.

137. **signs of an anxiety disorder:** "Anxiety Disorders." National Institute of Mental Health, April 2022; https://www.nimh.nih.gov/health/topics/anxiety-disorders.

137. **Depression, meanwhile, can feel like a sadness:** "Depression in Women: 5 Things You Should Know." National Institute of Mental Health, 2020; https://www.nimh.nih.gov/health/publications/depression-in-women.

139. **Research published in 2018 in *Socius*:** Daniel L. Carlson, Amanda Jayne Miller, and Sharon Sassler, "Stalled for Whom? Change in the Division of Particular Housework Tasks and Their Consequences for Middle- to Low-Income Couples." *Socius: Sociological Research for a Dynamic World* 4 (2018); doi: 10.1177/2378023118765867.

140. **"I suffered brain fog and anxiety":** Claire Toureille, "Davina McCall Says She Feared She Had a 'Brain Tumour or Alzheimer's' after Menopause Symptoms Caused Her to Make a Mistake on TV—And Admits She Felt 'Aged' and 'Embarrassed.'" *Daily Mail*, May 1, 2022; https://www.dailymail.co.uk/femail/article-10772431/Davina-McCall-reveals-thought-menopause-symptoms-brain-tumour.html.

144. **Perimenopause WTF?!:** Perry, "Perimenopause WTF?!—Your Perimenopause Sisterhood." Facebook group, August 2, 2019; https://www.facebook.com/groups/heyperry/about/.

144. **NAMS does *not* recommend menopausal hormone therapy:** NAMS 2017 Hormone Therapy Position Statement Advisory Panel, "The 2017 Hormone Therapy Position Statement of the North American Menopause Society." *Menopause* 24, no. 7 (2017): 728–53; doi: 10.1097/GME.0000000000000921.

145. **"you're not quite sure who you are anymore":** hey tim honey, "Jane Fonda on Oprah Winfrey 27.10.2010." YouTube, November 7, 2018, 2:09; https://www.youtube.com/watch?v=-NWS9zM-mW8.

146. **A meta-analysis of twenty-five randomized clinical trials:** Felipe B. Schuch et al., "Exercise as a Treatment for Depression: A Meta-Analysis Adjusting for Publication Bias." *Journal of Psychiatric Research* 77 (2016): 42–51; doi: 10.1016/j.jpsychires.2016.02.023.

146. **"Our entire physiology was designed":** Kelly McGonigal, *The Joy of Movement: How Exercise Helps Us Find Happiness, Hope, Connection, and Courage* (New York: Avery, 2021), 5–6.

146. **temptation bundling:** Katherine L. Milkman, Julia A. Minson, and Kevin G. M. Volpp, "Holding the Hunger Games Hostage at the Gym: An Evaluation of

Temptation Bundling." *Management Science* 60, no. 2 (2014): 283–99; doi: 10.1287/mnsc.2013.1784.

147. **menopausal women who listened to music:** Derya Yüksel Koçak and Yeliz Varişoğlu, "The Effect of Music Therapy on Menopausal Symptoms and Depression: A Randomized-Controlled Study." *Menopause* 29, no. 5 (2022): 545–52; doi: 10.1097/GME.0000000000001941.

CHAPTER 8: THE DRY VAGINA MONOLOGUES

149. **In 2014, it was renamed as the less-depressing:** Kyveli Angelou et al., "The Genitourinary Syndrome of Menopause: An Overview of the Recent Data." *Cureus* 12, no. 4 (2020): e7586; doi: 10.7759/cureus.7586.
149. **GSM, which afflicts a multitude of postmenopausal women:** Angelou et al., "The Genitourinary Syndrome of Menopause: An Overview of the Recent Data."
150. **skin that becomes markedly less supple, drier:** Mayo Clinic Staff, "Vaginal Atrophy." Mayo Clinic, September 17, 2021; https://www.mayoclinic.org/diseases-conditions/vaginal-atrophy/symptoms-causes/syc-20352288.
150. **a 2020 overview of GSM in the medical journal *Cureus*:** Angelou et al., "The Genitourinary Syndrome of Menopause: An Overview of the Recent Data."
151. **episodes of urine leakage:** North American Menopause Society, *The Menopause Guidebook,* 9th ed. (Pepper Pike, OH, 2020), 17.
152. **"avoidance of sexual situations":** Maria Uloko and Rachel Rubin, "Managing Female Sexual Pain." *Urologic Clinics of North America* 48, no. 4 (2021): 487–97; doi: 10.1016/j.ucl.2021.06.007.
153. **"People have the wrong assumption":** Gavanndra Hodge, "Interview: Salma Hayek: 'I Am a Lot More Than What You See.'" *The Sunday Times,* June 27, 2021; https://www.thetimes.co.uk/article/salma-hayek-i-am-a-lot-more-than-what-you-see-glv6c3ndw.
154. **not a recognized disorder until 2013:** Anna-Carlotta Zarski, Matthias Berking, and David Daniel Ebert, "Efficacy of Internet-Based Guided Treatment for Genito-Pelvic Pain/Penetration Disorder: Rationale, Treatment Protocol, and Design of a Randomized Controlled Trial." *Frontiers in Psychiatry* 8 (2018): 260; doi: 10.3389/fpsyt.2017.00260.
154. **up to 45 percent of postmenopausal women find sex painful:** "Pain with Penetration." North American Menopause Society, accessed July 9, 2022; https://www.menopause.org/for-women/sexual-health-menopause-online/sexual-problems-at-midlife/pain-with-penetration.

155. **GSM can be clinically detected:** S. Palacios et al., EVES Study Investigators, "The European Vulvovaginal Epidemiological Survey (EVES): Prevalence, Symptoms and Impact of Vulvovaginal Atrophy of Menopause." *Climacteric* 21, no. 3 (2018): 286–91; doi: 10.1080/13697137.2018.1446930.

155. **first line of treatment for GSM:** David D. Rahn et al., "Vaginal Estrogen for Genitourinary Syndrome of Menopause." *Obstetrics and Gynecology* 124, no. 6 (2014): 1147–56; doi: 10.1097/AOG.0000000000000526.

156. **amount of estrogen absorbed:** Megan Krause et al., "Local Effects of Vaginally Administered Estrogen Therapy: A Review." *Journal of Pelvic Medicine and Surgery* 15, no. 3 (2009): 105–14; doi: 10.1097/SPV.0b013e3181ab4804.

156. **A 2018 analysis of data from the Women's Health Initiative:** Carolyn J. Crandall et al., "Breast Cancer, Endometrial Cancer, and Cardiovascular Events in Participants Who Used Vaginal Estrogen in the Women's Health Initiative Observational Study." *Menopause* 25, no. 1 (2018): 11–20; doi: 10.1097/GME.00000 00000000956.

156. **2020 study concluded that vaginal estrogen:** Laura M. Chambers et al., "Vaginal Estrogen Use for Genitourinary Symptoms in Women with a History of Uterine, Cervical, or Ovarian Carcinoma." *International Journal of Gynecological Cancer* 30, no. 4 (2020): 515–24; doi: 10.1136/ijgc-2019-001034.

156. **In a 2014 review of forty-four studies:** David D. Rahn et al., "Vaginal Estrogen for Genitourinary Syndrome of Menopause: A Systemic Review." *Obstetrics and Gynecology* 124, no. 6 (2014): 1147–56; doi: 10.1097/AOG.0000000000000526.

156. **in the journal *Female Pelvic Medicine & Reconstructive Surgery*:** Eric Chang et al., "Vaginal Estrogen as First-Line Therapy for Recurrent Urinary Tract Infections in Postmenopausal Women and Risk Factors for Needing Additional Therapy." *Female Pelvic Medicine & Reconstructive Surgery* 27, no. 3 (2021): e487–e492; doi: 10.1097/SPV.0000000000000989.

157. **"As the research currently stands," announces the National Women's Health Network:** "Menopause." National Women's Health Network, accessed July 9, 2022; https://nwhn.org/issues/menopause/.

157–158. **have been lobbying the FDA to get rid of what Santoro calls:** JoAnn V. Pinkerton et al., "Workshop on Normal Reference Ranges for Estradiol in Postmenopausal Women: Commentary from the North American Menopause Society on Low-Dose Vaginal Estrogen Therapy Labeling." *Menopause* 27, no. 6 (2020):611–13; doi: 10.1097/GME.0000000000001576.

159. **Ospemifene has been shown:** Jae Jun Shin et al., "Ospemifene: A Novel Option for the Treatment of Vulvovaginal Atrophy." *Journal of Menopausal Medicine* 23, no. 2 (2017): 79–84; doi: 10.6118/jmm.2017.23.2.79.

159. **DHEA (dehydroepiandrosterone), meanwhile, is a hormone that metabolizes:**

Céline Martel et al., "Serum Steroid Concentrations Remain Within Normal Postmenopausal Values in Women Receiving Daily 6.5MG Intravaginal Prasterone for 12 Weeks." *Journal of Steroid Biochemistry and Molecular Biology* 159 (March 2016): 142–53; doi: 10.1016/j.jsbmb.2016.03.016.

159. **Laser therapy:** JoAnn V. Pinkerton, "FDA Mandating Vaginal Laser Manufacturers Present Valid Data Before Marketing." North American Menopause Society, August 1, 2018; https://www.menopause.org/docs/default-source/default-document-library/nams-responds-to-fda-mandate-on-vaginal-laser-manufacturers-08-01-2018.pdf.

159. **when basic measures fail:** North American Menopause Society, *The Menopause Guidebook,* 9th ed., 20.

159. **masturbation as a remedy:** "When Sex Is Painful." American College of Obstetricians and Gynecologists, January 2022; https://www.acog.org/womens-health/faqs/when-sex-is-painful.

161. **these lubricants on Facebook:** Valeriya Safronova, "Why Did Facebook Reject These Ads?" *New York Times,* January 11, 2022; https://www.nytimes.com/2022/01/11/style/facebook-womens-sexual-health-advertising.html.

161. **the medical journal *Maturitas*:** Alicia L. Muhleisen and Melissa M. Herbst-Kralovetz, "Menopause and the Vaginal Microbiome." *Maturitas* 91 (2016): 42–50; doi: 10.1016/j.maturitas.2016.05.015.

163. **"women give up the idea of sex":** Joanna Moorhead, "Interview: Marina Abramović: 'I Think About Dying Every Day.'" *The Guardian*, September 25, 2021; https://www.theguardian.com/artanddesign/2021/sep/25/this-much-i-know-marina-abramovic-i-think-about-dying-every-day-to-fully-enjoy-life.

164. **the National Association for Continence:** "Why You Shouldn't Use a Maxi-Pad for Incontinence." Bhealth Blog, accessed July 9, 2022; https://www.nafc.org/bhealth-blog/why-you-shouldnt-use-a-maxi-pad-for-incontinence.

CHAPTER 9: HORMONE THERAPY—LET'S GO THERE

169. **In 2021, an Indiana urogynecologist:** Ryan Stewart (stuboo), "I have the opportunity to design my office from scratch." Twitter, December 5, 2021; https://twitter.com/stuboo/status/1467522852664532994.

170. **no longer called hormone replacement therapy:** Christie Aschwanden, "Hormone Therapy, Long Shunned for a Possible Breast Cancer Link, Is Now Seen as a Short-Term Treatment for Menopause Symptoms." *Washington Post*, February 29, 2020; https://www.washingtonpost.com/health/hormone-therapy-long-shunned-for-a-possible-breast-cancer-link-is-now-seen-as-safe-and-helpful

-as-a-short-term-treatment-for-most-women-in-the-throes-of-menopause/2020/02/28/1fd19f66-54cd-11ea-929a-64efa7482a77_story.html.

171. **MHT is used to treat common symptoms:** "Hormone Therapy for Menopause Symptoms." Cleveland Clinic, June 28, 2021; https://my.clevelandclinic.org/health/treatments/15245-hormone-therapy-for-menopause-symptoms.

171. **the Women's Health Initiative, an unusually large long-term national health study:** Angelo Cagnacci and Martina Venier, "The Controversial History of Hormone Replacement Therapy." *Medicina* 55, no. 9 (2019): 602; doi: 10.3390/medicina55090602.

172. **plummeted by half:** Cagnacci and Venier, "The Controversial History of Hormone Replacement Therapy."

172. **animal activist groups:** People for the Ethical Treatment of Animals, "Premarin: A Prescription for Cruelty." PETA; https://www.peta.org/issues/animals-used-for-experimentation/animals-used-experimentation-factsheets/premarin-prescription-cruelty/.

172. **sarcophagus was pried open:** Judith A. Houck, "'What Do These Women Want?': Feminist Responses to *Feminine Forever*, 1963–1980." *Bulletin of the History of Medicine* 77, no. 1 (2003): 103–32; https://www.jstor.org/stable/44447695.

172. **Wilson had apparently accepted funds:** Ellen Goodman, "So Much for Hormone 'Salvation.'" *Washington Post*, July 13, 2002; https://www.washingtonpost.com/archive/opinions/2002/07/13/so-much-for-hormone-salvation/a80ec9ec-6219-4008-9f8f-90384af2f672/?itid=lk_inline_manual_6.

172. **Premarin was the fifth-most-prescribed drug:** Grace E. Kohn et al., "The History of Estrogen Therapy." *Sexual Medicine Reviews* 7, no. 3 (2019): 416–21; doi: 10.1016/j.sxmr.2019.03.006.

172. **MHT's reputation took a hit:** Kohn et al., "The History of Estrogen Therapy."

173. **"Having that hormone support":** Trinny Woodall, "Let's Talk Menopause." Facebook video, October 4, 2020, 6:02; https://www.facebook.com/watch/?v=335748134178781.

174. **The average age of participants in the WHI:** Rebecca C. Chester, Juliana M. Kling, and JoAnn E. Manson, "What the Women's Health Initiative Has Taught Us About Menopausal Hormone Therapy." *Clinical Cardiology* 41, no. 2 (2018): 247–52; doi: 10.1002/clc.22891.

174. **A reanalysis of the WHI trial:** Eric Roehm, "A Reappraisal of Women's Health Initiative Estrogen-Alone Trial: Long-Term Outcomes in Women 50–59 Years of Age," *Obstetrics and Gynecology International* 7 (2015): 713295; doi: 10.1155/2015/713295.

174. **Manson wrote in the journal *Women's Health*:** JoAnn Manson, "The Women's Health Initiative: The Latest Findings from Long-Term Follow-Up." *Women's Health* 10, no. 2 (2014): 125–28; doi: 10.2217/whe.14.6.

175. **critical window hypothesis:** Pauline M. Maki, "The Critical Window Hypothesis of Hormone Therapy and Cognition: A Scientific Update on Clinical Studies." *Menopause* 20, no. 6 (2013): 695–709; doi: 10.1097/GME.0b013e3182960cf8.

175. ***American Journal of Physiology: Heart and Circulatory Physiology*:** Robert C. Speth et al., "A Heartfelt Message, Estrogen Replacement Therapy: Use It or Lose It." *American Journal of Physiology* 315, no. 6 (2018): H1765–H1778; doi: 10.1152/ajpheart.00041.2018.

175. **NAMS's position statement on MHT:** North American Menopause Society, "The 2017 Hormone Therapy Position Statement of the North American Menopause Society." *Menopause* 24, no. 7 (2017): 728–53, doi: 10.1097/GME.0000000000000921.

176. **"wine at dinner nightly":** Sharon Malone and Jennifer Weiss-Wolf, "Opinion: America Lost Its Way on Menopause Research. It's Time to Get Back on Track." *Washington Post,* April 28, 2022; https://www.washingtonpost.com/opinions/2022/04/28/menopause-hormone-therapy-nih-went-wrong/.

177. **factors to help you in your decision:** "Hormone Therapy for Menopause Symptoms." Cleveland Clinic, June 28, 2021; https://my.clevelandclinic.org/health/treatments/15245-hormone-therapy-for-menopause-symptoms.

177. **If you're considering MHT, have your doctor take:** "Facts About Menopausal Hormone Therapy." U.S. Department of Health and Human Services, June 2005; https://www.nhlbi.nih.gov/files/docs/pht_facts.pdf.

177. **The amount and potency of hormones:** "Menopause Guide." WebMD, accessed July 9, 2022; https://www.webmd.com/menopause/guide/default.htm.

177–178. **ACOG's website maintains that transdermal therapy:** Committee on Gynecologic Practice, "Postmenopausal Estrogen Therapy Route of Administration and Risk of Venous Thromboembolism." American College of Obstetricians and Gynecologists, Number 556, April 2013; https://www.acog.org/clinical/clinical-guidance/committee-opinion/articles/2013/04/postmenopausal-estrogen-therapy-route-of-administration-and-risk-of-venous-thromboembolism.

178. **"Avoid fire, flame":** "Relief for Moderate-to-Severe Hot Flashes." Evamist, accessed July 9, 2022; https://evamist.com.

178. **If you've had your uterus removed:** R. Morgan Griffin, "Surgical Menopause: Should You Take Estrogen after Your Hysterectomy?" WebMD, June 21, 2020; https://www.webmd.com/menopause/guide/surgical-menopause-estrogen-after-hysterectomy.

178. **an oral contraceptive pill can manage:** Moon Kyoung Cho, "Use of Combined Oral Contraceptives in Perimenopausal Women." *Chonnam Medical Journal* 54, no. 3 (2018): 153–58; doi: 10.4068/cmj.2018.54.3.153.

178–179. **according to government data from 2020:** National Center for Health Statistics, "Contraceptive Use." Centers for Disease Control and Prevention, November 10, 2020; https://www.cdc.gov/nchs/fastats/contraceptive.htm.

180. **a 2022 study:** Haim A. Abenhaim et al., "Menopausal Hormone Therapy Formulation and Breast Cancer Risk." *Obstetrics & Gynecology* 139, no. 6 (2022): 1103–10; doi: 10.1097/AOG.0000000000004723.

180. **according to a 2019 editorial:** Louise Newson and Janice Rymer, "The Dangers of Compounded Bioidentical Hormone Replacement Therapy." *British Journal of General Practice* 69, no. 688 (2019): 540–41; doi: https://doi.org/10.3399/bjgp 19X706169.

180. **Chronic sleep loss over time:** Committee on Sleep Medicine and Research, "Extent and Health Consequences of Chronic Sleep Loss and Sleep Disorders," in *Sleep Disorders and Sleep Deprivation: An Unmet Public Health Problem,* Harvey R. Colten and Bruce M. Altevogt, eds. (Washington, DC: National Academies Press, 2006); https://www.ncbi.nlm.nih.gov/books/NBK19960/.

182. **the journal *Science Translational Medicine*:** Slavenka Kam-Hansen et al., "Altered Placebo and Drug Labeling Changes the Outcome of Episodic Migraine Attacks." *Science Translational Medicine* 6, no. 218 (2014): 218ra5; doi: 10.1126/scitranslmed.3006175.

183. ***Bioidentical* refers to compounds:** Newton and Rymer, "The Dangers of Compounded Bioidentical Hormone Replacement Therapy."

183. **Instead of being manufactured by a multinational:** "What Is Custom-Compounded Therapy?" North American Menopause Society, accessed July 9, 2022; https://www.menopause.org/publications/clinical-practice-materials/bio identical-hormone-therapy/what-is-custom-compounded-therapy-.

184. **"[Menopause] is as natural":** Elizabeth Narins, "Kim Cattrall Imagines the *Sex and the City* Cast Going Through Menopause." *Cosmopolitan*, September 24, 2014; https://www.cosmopolitan.com/entertainment/interviews/a31451/kim-cat trall-menopause-interview/.

185. **a 2015 NAMS survey revealed:** North American Menopause Society, "Use of Compounded Hormone Therapy in the United States: Report of the North American Menopause Society Survey." *Menopause* 22, no. 12 (2015): 1276–84; https://www.menopause.org/docs/default-source/professional/use-of-com pounded-hormone-therapy-survey.pdf?sfvrsn=2.

185. **a 2017 review in the journal *Climacteric*:** M. L'Hermite, "Custom-Compounded Bioidentical Hormone Therapy: Why So Popular Despite Potential Harm? The Case Against Routine Use." *Climacteric* 20, no. 3 (2017): 205–11; doi: 10.1080/13697137.2017.1285277.

185. **a 2020 report issued by the National Academies:** "Prescribers Should Restrict the Use of Non-FDA-Approved Compounded Bioidentical Hormones, Except

for Specific Medical Circumstances." National Academies of Science, Engineering, and Medicine, July 1, 2020; https://www.nationalacademies.org/news/2020/07/prescribers-should-restrict-the-use-of-non-fda-approved-compounded-bioidentical-hormones-except-for-specific-medical-circumstances.

185. **As NAMS points out on its website:** "Menopause FAQS: Hormone Therapy for Menopause Symptoms." North American Menopause Society, accessed July 9, 2022; https://www.menopause.org/for-women/menopause-faqs-hormone-therapy-for-menopause-symptoms.

185. **In 2013, *More* magazine did a now-famous investigation:** Cathryn Jakobson Ramin, "The Hormone Hoax Thousands Fall For." *More,* October 2013; https://www.menopause.org/docs/default-source/professional/the-hormone-hoax-thousands-fall-for-oct-2013-more.pdf.

186. **Compounding pharmacies can be useful for several reasons:** National Academies of Sciences, Engineering, and Medicine, "The Use of Compounded Bioidentical Hormone Therapy," in *The Clinical Utility of Compounded Bioidentical Hormone Therapy: A Review of Safety, Effectiveness, and Use,* L. M. Jackson, R. M. Parker, and D. R. Mattison, eds. (Washington, DC: National Academies Press, 2020); https://www.ncbi.nlm.nih.gov/books/NBK562886/.

188. **Testosterone therapy:** Streicher, *Hot Flash Hell,* 208.

189. **the UK faced an acute shortage:** "Menopause: HRT Rationed amid Continuing Shortage in UK." BBC News, April 29, 2022; https://www.bbc.com/news/health-61278325.

189. **An estimated one million women:** "Menopause: Diagnosis and Management." National Institute for Health and Care Excellence, November 12, 2015; https://www.nice.org.uk/guidance/ng23/chapter/context.

189. **total number of females is around 33 million:** Office for National Statistics, "Overview of the UK Population: January 2021." January 14, 2021; https://www.ons.gov.uk/peoplepopulationandcommunity/populationandmigration/populationestimates/articles/overviewoftheukpopulation/january2021.

189. **"become drug mules":** Xantha Leatham and Sophie Huskisson, "Shortage of HRT May Force Women to Become Drug Mules by Travelling Overseas to Buy Vital Supplies of Medication, Experts Warn." *Daily Mail,* April 26, 2022; https://www.dailymail.co.uk/news/article-10756739/HRT-shortage-Women-drug-mules-travelling-overseas-experts-warn.html.

189. **One woman called thirty pharmacies:** Sarah Graham, "HRT Shortage Explained: Desperate Ways Women Are Dealing with the Menopause and What Caused the Crisis." *inews,* May 4, 2022; https://inews.co.uk/news/health/hrt-shortage-explained-desperate-women-dealing-menopause-cause-1608789.

189. **"Meeting in a car park":** Mariella Frostrup, "Why Ending This HRT Crisis Really Is a Matter of Life or Death for Women." *Daily Mail,* April 25, 2022;

https://www.dailymail.co.uk/debate/article-10752561/The-shortage-menopause-drugs-isnt-niche-feminist-issue-argues-MARIELLA-FROSTRUP.html.

190. **Some women reported that they felt suicidal:** Maya Oppenheim, "HRT Shortage Leaving Menopausal Women Suicidal and Causing Relationship Breakdowns, MP Warns." *The Independent,* April 22, 2022; https://www.independent.co.uk/news/uk/home-news/hrt-shortage-menopause-relationship-breakdown-b2063416.html.

190. **appointed an MHT tsar:** Department of Health and Social Care, Maria Caulfield, and Sajid Javid, "Vaccine Taskforce Director General Will Harness Lessons from Pandemic to Address HRT Supply Chain Issues." Gov.uk, April 29, 2022; https://www.gov.uk/government/news/vaccine-taskforce-director-general-will-harness-lessons-from-pandemic-to-address-hrt-supply-chain-issues.

CHAPTER 10: THE RESTORATION

194. **In a 2008 study published in the journal *Health Care for Women International*:** María Luisa Marván et al., "Stereotypes of Women in Different Stages of Their Reproductive Life: Data from Mexico and the United States." *Health Care for Women International* 29, no. 7 (2008): 673–87; doi: 10.1080/07399330802188982.

194. **2022 study in the *Journal of Women & Aging*:** Vanessa Cecil et al., "Gendered Ageism and Gray Hair: Must Older Women Choose Between Feeling Authentic and Looking Competent?" *Journal of Women & Aging* 34, no. 2 (2022): 210–25; doi: 10.1080/08952841.2021.1899744.

195. **"I'm going through perimenopause":** Sabrina Park, "Tracee Ellis Ross Isn't Afraid to Talk About Aging." *Harper's Bazaar,* November 1, 2021, https://www.harpersbazaar.com/celebrity/latest/a38092624/tracee-ellis-ross-isnt-afraid-to-talk-about-aging/.

196. **In a 2010 review in the journal *Maturitas*:** Beverley Ayers, Mark Forshaw, and Myra S. Hunter, "The Impact of Attitudes Towards the Menopause on Women's Symptom Experience: A Systematic Review." *Maturitas* 65, no. 1 (2010): 28–36; doi: 10.1016/j.maturitas.2009.10.016.

196. **men about perimenopause and menopause:** *Health* magazine, "7 Men Answer Questions on Menopause | Health." YouTube, December 1, 2017, 1:07; https://www.youtube.com/watch?v=DtH2OKCP9UM.

201. **forget the ad for the GLH System:** Coolestmovies, "1990's Infomercial Hell #19: 'The Babes Are Back' with Ron Popeil's GLH Canned Hair, by Ronco!" YouTube, 2:00; https://www.youtube.com/watch?v=2GeF7A05zQ8.

204. **Ulta, the nation's largest beauty retailer:** "Womaness Becomes First Modern Menopause Brand to Enter Ulta Beauty." Cision PR Newswire, May 16, 2022; https://www.prnewswire.com/news-releases/womaness-becomes-first-modern-menopause-brand-to-enter-ulta-beauty-301545485.html.

204. **only 7.2 percent:** Dongqing Wang et al., "Healthy Lifestyle During the Midlife Is Prospectively Associated with Less Subclinical Carotid Atherosclerosis: The Study of Women's Health Across the Nation." *Journal of the American Heart Association* 7, no. 23 (2018): e010405; doi: 10.1161/JAHA.118.010405.

204. **the latest physical activity guidelines from the U.S. Department of Health:** U.S. Department of Health and Human Services, *Physical Activity Guidelines for Americans, 2nd Edition* (Washington, DC: U.S. Department of Health and Human Services, 2018); https://health.gov/sites/default/files/2019-09/Physical_Activity_Guidelines_2nd_edition.pdf.

205. **The Endocrine Society's website warns that menopause:** "Menopause and Bone Loss." Endocrine Society, January 24, 2022; https://www.endocrine.org/patient-engagement/endocrine-library/menopause-and-bone-loss.

205. **A 2010 meta-analysis in the journal *Medicine & Science in Sports & Exercise*:** Mark D. Peterson et al., "Resistance Exercise for Muscular Strength in Older Adults: A Meta-Analysis." *Ageing Research Review* 9, no. 3 (2010): 226–37; doi: 10.1016/j.arr.2010.03.004.

205. **Strength training (or even weight-bearing aerobic exercises):** "Strength Training Builds More Than Muscle." Harvard Health Publishing, October 13, 2021; https://www.health.harvard.edu/staying-healthy/strength-training-builds-more-than-muscles.

205. **The simple act of jumping up and down:** J. Eric Strong, "Effects of Different Jumping Programs on Hip and Spine Bone Mineral Density in Pre-Menopausal Women" (PhD dissertation, Brigham Young University, 2004).

207. **"Menopause has been a taboo subject":** Some Like it HOTT Podcast, "Menopause has been a taboo subject for far too long." Facebook video, May 6, 2021, 0:29; https://m.facebook.com/watch/?v=133279992152289&_rdr.

208. **In 2022, a group even sprang up:** The Kingfisher, "Mother and Daughter Start Menopause Support Group in Ipswich." Facebook post, May 10, 2022; https://z-upload.facebook.com/kingfisherpub/posts/10158373627562536.

208. **as Dr. Nanette Santoro wrote:** Nanette Santoro, C. Neill Epperson, and Sarah B. Mathews, "Menopausal Symptoms and Their Management." *Endocrinology & Metabolism Clinics of North America* 44, no. 3 (2015): 497–515; doi: 10.1016/j.ecl.2015.05.001.

CONCLUSION: MENO-POSITIVITY!

213. **spat back into the bottle:** Court of Appeal of Louisiana, Second Circuit, *Hollis v. Ouachita Coca-Cola Bottling Co., Limited,* No. 6128, May 3, 1940; https://casetext.com/case/hollis-v-ouachita-coca-cola-bottling-co.
214. **Anna Laskowski was knocked down:** Michigan Supreme Court, *Laskowski v. People's Ice Co.,* 203 Mich. 186 (2 A.L.R. 586).
214. **"menopause defense":** Phyllis T. Bookspan and Maxine Kline, "On Mirror and Gavels: A Chronicle of How Menopause Was Used as a Legal Defense Against Women." *Indiana Law Review* 32, no. 4 (1999): 1267–1334; https://journals.iupui.edu/index.php/inlawrev/article/view/3382/3311.
215. **"Menopause is an age of opportunity":** Kristen Baldwin, "Cynthia Nixon on Miranda's *And Just Like That* Journey: 'Menopause Gets a Bad Rap.'" *Entertainment Weekly,* December 22, 2020; https://ew.com/tv/miranda-and-just-like-that-cynthia-nixon.
216. **four-nation Menopause Taskforce:** Department of Health and Social Care, "Nation Unite to Tackle Menopause Taskforce." Gov.uk, February 3, 2022; https://www.gov.uk/government/news/nations-unite-to-tackle-menopause-taskforce.
216. **Children are learning about menopause in England's schools:** Department for Education, "Relationships and Sex Education (RSE) (Secondary)." Gov.uk, September 13, 2021; https://www.gov.uk/government/publications/relationships-education-relationships-and-sex-education-rse-and-health-education/relationships-and-sex-education-rse-secondary.
216. **UK's Menopause Workplace Pledge:** "Menopause Workplace Pledge." Well-Being of Women, accessed July 9, 2022; https://www.wellbeingofwomen.org.uk/campaigns/menopausepledge.
217. **A 2022 survey by the UK's Fawcett Society:** "Menopause and the Workplace." Fawcett, accessed July 9, 2022; https://www.fawcettsociety.org.uk/menopauseandtheworkplace.
217. **In 2022, London's mayor Sadiq Khan:** "Mayor Announces World-Leading Menopause Policy." London.gov.uk, March 8, 2022; https://www.london.gov.uk/press-releases/mayoral/mayor-announces-world-leading-menopause-policy.
217. **"What we've got to do as blokes":** Lorraine, "Sadiq Khan on Removing the Menopause Taboo in the Workplace & Keeping Women Safe on the Streets | LK." YouTube, March 8, 2022, 1:13, https://www.youtube.com/watch?v=kx5eQL5aN04.
217. **A 2022 report from the UK organization Menopause Experts:** Yoana Cholteeva, "Employment Tribunals Citing Menopause up in 2021, Report Show." *People*

Management, June 1, 2022; https://www.peoplemanagement.co.uk/article/1788405/employment-tribunals-citing-menopause-2021-report-shows.

218. **"Support Menopause, or Prepare for Court":** Jonathan Ames, "Support Menopause or Prepare for Court, Firms Told." *The Sunday Times*, November 28, 2011; https://www.thetimes.co.uk/article/support-menopause-or-prepare-for-court-firms-told-vczgqq75z.

218. **the Nottingham-based organization Henpicked:** Henpicked, 11 High Street, Ruddington, Nottingham NG11 6DT; https://henpicked.net/about-us.

218. **In Australia, more than $40 million:** "$40 Million in Funding for Menopause Services." NSW Government Treasury, June 10, 2022; https://www.treasury.nsw.gov.au/news/40-million-funding-menopause-services.

218. **"how difficult it can be":** Lucy Cormack, "$40.3M Funding Boost to Support Women Facing 'Debilitating' Reality of Menopause." *Sydney Morning Herald*, June 10, 2022; https://www.smh.com.au/politics/nsw/40-3m-funding-boost-to-support-women-facing-debilitating-reality-of-menopause-20220609-p5asn5.html.

218. **the Australian company Future Super:** Khaila (Khi) Prasser, "A Bloody Good Policy." Future Super, February 12, 2021; https://www.futuresuper.com.au/blog/a-bloody-good-policy.

218–219. **As a 2019 editorial in the *Journal of Management*:** Alicia A. Grandey, Allison S. Gabriel, and Eden B. King, "Tackling Taboo Topics: A Review of the Three *M*s in Working Women's Lives," *Journal of Management* 46, no. 1 (2019): 7–35; doi: 10.1177/0149206319857144.

219. **global productivity losses:** Lizzy Burden, "Women Are Leaving the Workforce for a Little-Talked-About Reason." *Bloomberg*, June 18, 2021; https://www.bloomberg.com/news/articles/2021-06-18/women-are-leaving-the-workforce-for-a-little-talked-about-reason#xj4y7vzkg.

219. **women make up nearly half of the workforce:** BLS Reports, "Women in the Labor Force: A Databook." U.S. Bureau of Labor Statistics, April 2021; https://www.bls.gov/opub/reports/womens-databook/2020/home.htm.

219. **The U.S.-based Let's Talk Menopause:** "Menopause and the Workplace." Let's Talk Menopause, accessed July 9, 2022; https://www.letstalkmenopause.org/menopause-and-the-workplace.

219. **ERGs, as *The Wall Street Journal* has reported:** Joann S. Lublin, "Employee Resource Groups Are on the Rise at U.S. Companies." *Wall Street Journal*, October 31, 2021; https://www.wsj.com/articles/why-ergs-are-on-the-rise-11635532232.

220. **"a time in your life when you get back to":** Shanti Escalante, "Emily Gould Is Looking Forward to Menopause." *Interview*, April 13, 2020; https://www.interviewmagazine.com/culture/emily-gould-perfect-tunes.

221. **around 35 percent of companies:** Tiffany Burns et al., "Women in the Workplace." McKinsey & Company, September 27, 2021; https://www.mckinsey.com/featured-insights/diversity-and-inclusion/women-in-the-workplace.

221. **90 percent of major employers:** Starla Trigg, "ERG: An Acronym You Should Know." TOPMBA, April 5, 2021; https://www.topmba.com/blog/erg-acronym-you-should-know.

221. **some changes in the workplace that you could promote:** "A Guide to Managing Menopause at Work." Chartered Institute of Personnel and Development, May 2021; https://www.cipd.co.uk/Images/line-manager-guide-to-menopause_tcm18-95174.pdf.

222. **NAMS president Stephanie Faubion told *Fortune* magazine:** Kells McPhillips, "How to Manage (And Normalize) Menopause at Work." *Fortune* Well, May 20, 2022; https://fortune.com/2022/05/20/how-to-manage-menopause-at-work/.

222. **"One of the greatest under-appreciated sources":** A. Pawlowski, "Why Older Women Will Rule the World." today.com, December 5, 2017, https://www.today.com/health/older-women-will-rule-world-we-live-longer-t119645?cid=public-rss_20171206.

222. **is estimated to swell to $22 billion:** "Menopause Market Size Worth $22.7 Billion by 2028 | CAGR: 5.7%: Grand View Research, Inc." Bloomberg, June 14, 2021, https://www.bloomberg.com/press-releases/2021-06-14/menopause-market-size-worth-22-7-billion-by-2028-cagr-5-7-grand-view-research-inc.

223. **Boots debuted a Menopause Support Hub:** Francesca Rice, "Boots' Menopause Hub Launches to Help You Find Solutions for All 40 Signs and Symptoms." Yahoo! Finance UK, October 18, 2021, https://uk.finance.yahoo.com/news/boots-menopause-hub-launches-help-114900720.html.

224. **backed the telehealth start-up Evernow:** Bhanvi Satija, "Gwyneth Paltrow, Cameron Diaz–Backed Evernow raises $28.5 mln." Reuters, April 6, 2022; https://www.reuters.com/business/healthcare-pharmaceuticals/gwyneth-paltrow-cameron-diaz-backed-evernow-raises-285-mln-2022-04-06/.

224. **A subscription includes unlimited access:** "Real Science for Real Menopause Symptoms." Evernow, 2022; https://www.evernow.com/.

224. **New York–based Gameto:** "Redefining Female Reproductive Identity." gameto, 2022; https://gametogen.com/.

225. **"the real moonshot":** Beth Kowitt, "This Biotech Startup Thinks It Can Delay Menopause by 15 Years. That Would Transform Women's Lives." *Fortune*, April 19, 2021; https://fortune.com/2021/04/19/celmatix-delay-menopause-womens-ovarian-health/.

225. **the majority of ob-gyns are now female:** "The Controversy over the Dwindling

Ranks of Male Ob-Gyns, Explained." Advisory Board, March 14, 2018; https://www.advisory.com/daily-briefing/2018/03/14/male-obgyn.

225. **more U.S. medical students were women:** Brendan Murphy, "Women in Medical Schools: Dig into Latest Record-Breaking Numbers." American Medical Association, September 29, 2021; https://www.ama-assn.org/education/medical-school-diversity/women-medical-schools-dig-latest-record-breaking-numbers.

226. **popular Danish political thriller *Borgen*:** Lisa Abend, "Danish Political Drama *Borgen* Is Back at Last, with a Fresh Take on Female Power." *Time,* June 3, 2022; https://time.com/6183816/borgen-season-4-netflix/.

226. ***The Change*, a revenge-fantasy thriller:** Kirsten Miller, *The Change* (New York: HarperCollins, 2022), https://www.harpercollins.com/products/the-change-kirsten-miller?variant=39715444719650.

227. **"Make connections, make friends":** Morrill, Hannah, "No Matter Where You Are in Life, Cameron Diaz Has Some Advice for You." *Women's Health*, March 10, 2016; https://www.womenshealthmag.com/life/a19934235/cameron-diaz-life-advice/.

229. **Practicing self-compassion has been shown:** Filip Raes, "Rumination and Worry as Mediators of the Relationship Between Self-Compassion and Depression and Anxiety." *Personality and Individual Differences* 48 (2010): 757–61; https://self-compassion.org/wp-content/uploads/publications/ruminationmediators.pdf.

229. **Rebecca Thurston of the University of Pittsburgh:** Rebecca C. Thurston et al., "Self-Compassion and Subclinical Cardiovascular Disease Among Midlife Women." *Health Psychology* 40, no. 11 (2011): 747–53; doi: 10.1037/hea0001137.

229. **A 2020 study of middle-aged teachers in Eritrea:** Helen Gebretatyos et al., "Effect of Health Education on Knowledge and Attitude of Menopause Among Middle-Age Teachers." *BMC Women's Health* 20, no. 1 (2020): 232; doi: 10.1186/s12905-020-01095-2.

230. **A 2010 Taiwanese study of women:** S. A. R. Syed Alwi, I. B. Brohi, and I. Awi, "Perception of Menopause Among Women of Sarawak, Malaysia." *BMC Women's Health* 21, no. 1 (2012): 77; doi: 10.1186/s12905-021-01230-7.

231. **As Nora Ephron wrote in *I Feel Bad About My Neck*:** Nora Ephron, *I Feel Bad About My Neck: And Other Thoughts on Being a Woman* (New York: Knopf, 2006), 7.

Index